Hair loss: the answers

SUSAN ALDRIDGE

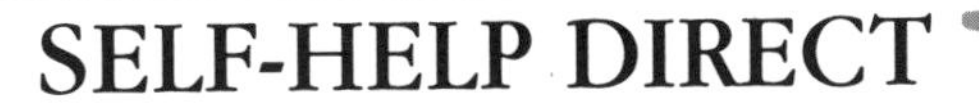

For more copies of this book, please send £10.95 cheque or postal order per book
(overseas sales $25 per book, postage & packing free) made payable to *Self-Help Direct* to:
Self-Help Direct Publishing
PO BOX 9035,
London, N12 8ED

DESIGN: Michael Crozier/Design Unlimited
COVER ILLUSTRATION: Michael Daley
GRAPHICS/ILLUSTRATIONS: Michael Roscoe

Published by Self-Help Direct Publishing, PO Box, London, N12 8ED
First edition 1997

ISBN 1 900461 10 2

contents

Acknowledgments

I am especially grateful to John Firmage and Dr Hugh Rushton for helpful discussions and for commenting upon parts of this book.

I would also like to thank Keith Hobbs, Philip Kingsley, Glenn Lyons, Bill Lennon, Michelle Goddard, Caroline Woolfson, Richard Mawbey, Dr Michael May, Andy Bryant, Deirdre Edwards, Annabel Fiddian-Green and Nigel Fawkes for their help and advice.

Finally, I would like to acknowledge all the people whose case histories appear here for sharing their experiences of hair loss with me.

About the author

Susan Aldridge has a PhD in chemistry and an MSc in biotechnology. Before taking up journalism, she worked for several years as a chemist for the Medical Research Council and has contributed to many research papers. Since 1988, she has worked as a freelance journalist. Her articles have appeared in many newspapers and magazines including *New Scientist*, *Genetic Engineering News* and *The Guardian*. She has written three books on genetics and biochemistry. The most recent is *The Thread of Life* which was published by Cambridge University Press in 1996.

She is currently researching a book about pharmaceutical drugs and complementary medicine. Since 1994, she has been Medical Editor of the popular monthly science and technology magazine *Focus*.

introduction

In September 1996 I wrote a feature on hair loss in 'Focus' magazine. The response was surprising; I had never received so many letters and phone calls about an article from readers wanting to know more. One reader, aged 18, wrote saying he was "really desperate" about his hair loss and did not know where to start looking for help. I hope he reads this book and discovers some of the options open to him.

Hair loss is a curiously neglected problem. There are self-help groups for people with every medical condition you can think of, yet when it comes to alopecia support is hard to come by – even though it affects up to one in three people, men and women alike. Hair loss causes immense distress. At the extreme it can lead to suicide. In the course of researching this book I was lucky enough to meet many people who faced up to hair loss with courage, confidence, and acceptance. Yet even they said they would have their hair back if there was a sure fire solution to the problem. All of them complained that there just is not enough information available. There are few books on the subject which are not written by people with a vested interest. And there are many so-called "hair specialists" around whose sole aim is to prey on vulnerable people.

This book forms part of a series of health books published by *Self-Help Direct*. It is aimed at people who want to learn more about a particular problem or condition with a view to taking a positive attitude to dealing or coping with it. *Hair Loss* is a comprehensive, independent, and unbiased guide to the subject. It aims to explode a few myths, and offer real advice and help for men and women concerned about the loss of hair.

Table 1. How to find your way around this book

If you are reading this book, we assume you have a hair loss problem and are concerned about it. Read on!

	Chapter									
	1	2	3	4	5	6	7	8	9	10
For a basic understanding of hair	✓									
If you do not know the cause of your hair loss		✓			✓					
If you have been diagnosed and want to take action					✓					
If you are undergoing/about to undergo chemotherapy for cancer					✓					
If you are interested in natural solutions or complementary therapies									✓	
If you are worried about the social/ psychological impact of hair loss			✓							
If you have decided to accept your hair loss but want to look good				✓						
If you want a permanent solution							✓			
If you want to complain about hair loss treatment you have had					✓					
If you are thinking about wearing a hairpiece						✓				
If you are interested in medical/drug treatments								✓		
If you are interested in future developments										✓

Chapter One

What is hair?

Hair consists of threads of cells which contain the protein keratin. Like fingernails and toenails, the hair is considered to be an appendage of the skin. Hair cells are dead; that is why having your hair cut is not painful.

There are three types of hair. Babies start to develop a fine, downy hair called lanugo all over their bodies around the third month of pregnancy. While you may notice this hair on premature babies, usually most of it is lost before birth – leaving lanugo on only the scalp and eyebrow area.

By the time a baby is five or six months old, lanugo is replaced by coarser hair known as terminal hair. Most of the rest of the body becomes covered in a fine, almost invisible, type of hair called vellus.

At puberty sex hormones stimulate the growth of further terminal hair around the genitals and in the armpits. In addition, boys start to develop terminal hair on the chest and in the beard area.

Hair usually grows everywhere on the body, except on the palms, soles, lips, the tip of the penis, the nipples, and the lips of the vulva, which surround the vagina.

Hair under the microscope.

The part of a hair which is visible above the surface of the skin is called the shaft. The hair root is embedded in the skin, in a small pit called a follicle (Figure 1). The lower portion of the root thickens into an area called the bulb. Sometimes, when you pull out a hair, its bulb is visible as a tiny white swelling at the bottom of the hair. New hair cells are produced in a patch of tissue in the bulb known as the matrix. The bulb pushes inwards at its base forming an area called the hair papilla. This is well supplied with tiny blood vessels which bring nutrients to the growing hair.

The shape of the follicle affects the appearance of the hair. A round follicle gives straight hair, an oval one wavy hair, while people with curly hair have spiral follicles. All the body's hair follicles, around five million in total, are present at birth. It is not possible to develop new hair follicles in adult life.

Figure 1: A single hair and its follicle
Hair grows out of a tiny pit in the skin known as a hair follicle. New hairs are produced from the bulb area.

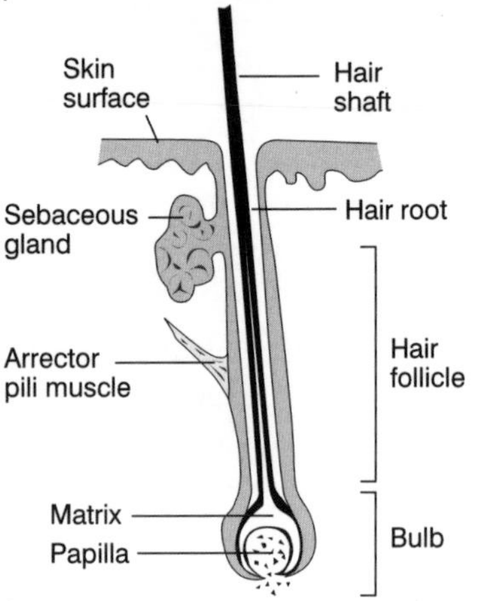

There are around 100,000 hair follicles on the scalp. For some unknown reason, the number of hairs on the head varies with hair colour. Blondes have most, with around 140,000 hairs, while dark-haired people have about 108,000. Redheads have the least, with only around 90,000 hairs.

The hair shaft normally grows at a angle to the skin; this provides more a effective protective coverage to the body.

However, the shaft is attached to a tiny muscle called the arrector pili, which can pull on the hair, pushing it up at right angles to the skin and creating a “goose bump”. This happens as an automatic reflex when the skin is exposed to low temperatures. The erect hairs trap a layer of insulating air close to the skin, in an attempt to stop the body losing heat.

The same response occurs when you are really scared (some

people feel the hairs at the back of their neck "stand on end").

The hair itself is made up of three layers (Figure 2). The inner medulla is composed of loosely packed cells containing soft keratin and has many air spaces. This is surrounded by the cortex, which is the thickest layer of the hair shaft. The cortex contains hard keratin as well as the pigments which give the hair its colour. Black, brown and fair hair contain varying concentrations of the dark pigment melanin. The colour of red hair comes from a different pigment called trichosiderin which, like blood and rust, contains iron. Over time, the cells in the cortex stop producing these pigments and so individual hairs turn white. Grey hair is actually a mixture of white hairs and hair of the original colour.

Figure 2: Section through the hair shaft

The hair shaft is composed of three layers: the innermost medulla, the cortex and the outer, thinnest layer, the cuticle

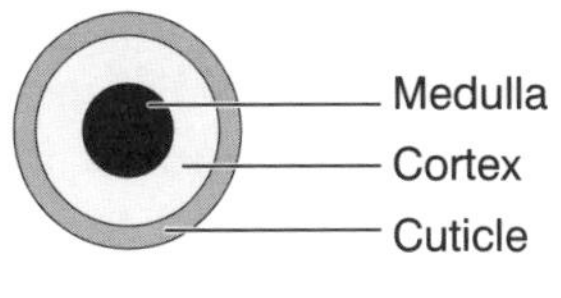

The outer layer of the hair, the cuticle, consists of layers of overlapping, scaly cells. The oil produced by the tiny sebaceous gland which is attached to the side of the hair follicle lubricates and protects the cuticle. However, cuticle cells may still be damaged by the over-use of hairdressing products such as bleaches, perms and colours, and can even be stripped off by harsh chemicals, such as the chlorine in swimming pool water.[2, 3, 4]

How hair grows

Hair has a growth cycle which is divided into three phases. The growth phase, known as anagen, lasts for on average from five to seven years. This is followed by a transition phase, catagen, of around two weeks during which the root of the hair becomes detached from the follicle and starts to move up towards the surface of the skin. Finally, the hair enters a rest phase, called telogen, which lasts for three to four months. The hair may be shed during this phase. If not, it will be pushed out by a new growing hair when the cycle begins again.

Each hair grows independently of the rest. At any one time 90 per cent of the 100,000 or so scalp hairs are in the anagen phase, with around one per cent being in transition and the rest in telogen, ready to be shed. It is quite normal to lose 50 to 100 hairs a day without the loss being at all apparent.

Scalp hair grows at a maximum rate of 0.4 millimetres a day, but this rate varies with age and time of the day and year.

If left uncut it would grow to a length of one metre in a lifetime. Any differences in length between male and female hair are cultural, rather than biological, in origin (remember the Sixties, when men showed they could have long hair too). Hair grows faster at night and in warmer weather. And coarse black hair appears to grow faster than fine blond hair. Shaving does not alter the rate of hair growth. In Britain hair loss peaks in August and September, because there are fewer follicles in the growing, or anagen, phase at this time of year.

The factors which affect the cycle of hair growth are not well understood, except that levels of thyroid hormones and of the sex hormones, oestrogen and testosterone, appear to play an important role.[2,3,4]

What is hair for?

Humans have longer scalp hair than any other primate species. As Desmond Morris points out in his book *Bodywatching*, our hair once served as an important species signal, setting us apart from other animals.[5]

Hair no longer has any survival value in humans, although it still does in other mammals. However, our hair still has a certain protective function. Scalp hair shields us from the sun and wind; the former is perhaps increasingly important in these days of ozone depletion, which exposes us to a higher intensity of damaging ultra-violet light. It also keeps us warm in cold weather – up to 25 per cent of body heat is lost through the head.

Hair on the head also gives some insulation against knocks and bumps. Eyebrows protect the eyes from sweat and the glare of the sun, while eyelashes provide a shield against dust and grit entering the eye. And the fine hairs that line the nostrils act as a filter, trapping dust and other particles. Similar protective hairs are found around the openings to other body organs such as the ears.

The condition of the hair is a useful 'barometer' of someone's state of health. Dry, brittle hair, for example, may indicate a problem with the thyroid gland. Hair analysis can also provide important diagnostic clues. Hair concentrates toxins such as arsenic and various drugs, including heroin and cocaine. Hair analysis is sometimes used by forensic experts to determine cause of death; it was used as long ago as 1910 to convict Dr Hawley Crippen of poisoning his wife with arsenic. It is also used as a sensitive measure of environmental pollution, while some health practitioners also use hair analysis in the diagnosis of mineral deficiencies.

However, the main significance of human hair today is as a means of sexual and social communication. A full head of hair, in both men and women, is associated with youth and attractiveness, especially if it is in tip-top condition. We spend millions of pounds a year on shampoos, conditioners, and other hair cosmetics, and even more on visits to the hairdresser.

At puberty, the appearance of pubic and underarm hair is a sign of sexual maturity. This body hair may also help in the dispersal of body odour, which is thought to contain sex attractants known as pheremones. In some cultures, beards are a sign of manhood.

Hair may also have cultural or religious significance. Over the course of human history, long hair in men has been considered as a symbol of strength and power. The words Caesar, Kaiser and Tsar all mean 'hairy' in their original form. In the Bible, Samson's legendary strength came from his hair and was lost when it was cut by Delilah. Male Sikhs do not cut their hair, because they too regard it as a natural symbol of strength, like a lion's mane. The Sikhs keep their long hair concealed beneath a turban, while Rastafarians display theirs in characteristic dreadlocks.

However, customs vary; St Paul said that men should have short hair, and women long hair – a ruling which persists in many societies today, with long-haired men being regarded as effeminate. And a shaved head in a woman was long considered a mark of shame. In Paris, for example, at the close of World War II, women suspected of sleeping with Germans had their heads shaved and were paraded through the streets as a punishment. On the other hand, a shaved head is the norm among women of the Masai and Dinka tribes in Africa. Nuns and Buddhist priests also shave their heads, as an outward symbol of their vows of chastity.

Women have often been required to keep their hair covered. For example, traditionally it is considered immodest for a Jewish married woman to appear in public with her head uncovered. Today many Orthodox Jewish women shave off their hair when they marry and wear a wig, known as a sheitel, to cover their heads when they go out.

Chapter 2

Hair loss

Hair loss can affect men or women of any age, at any time. The clinical term for hair loss is alopecia. In men, alopecia is commonly due to a combination of genetic and hormonal factors which leads to the common condition known as male pattern baldness or alopecia androgenetica. In this type of hair loss, the follicles are oversensitive to the male sex hormone (or androgen) known as dihydrotestosterone (DHT). Two thirds of all men will eventually be affected by this type of hair loss.

In women, genetic hair loss is less common, although the incidence increases markedly with age. While 10 per cent of women notice some hair loss in their thirties, this figure increases to 40 % for post-menopausal women. Fifty per cent of hair loss in women is genetic; the rest is caused by other hormone imbalances, stress, drugs, dieting, immune system disorders, or damage to the hair. Taking all these causes into account, women probably suffer from hair loss as much as men do.[3, 9, 10, 11]

Genetic hair loss

(also known as male or female pattern baldness, androgen-dependent alopecia, alopecia androgenetica, or common baldness).

By the time they reach their thirties, many men notice that they appear to be losing their hair. Each time a hair is shed, its replacement becomes progressively thinner. The overall effect is decreased coverage of the scalp. It may start as early as the teens or twenties, and is often a very gradual process.

Some men are only aware of balding when they look at recent holiday photos and compare them with snaps taken in the past.

Premature hair loss may start as early as the teens. What is happening is not so much increased shedding as progressive thinning. Finally the follicle stops producing hair altogether.

In genetic hair loss, which affects 7.4 million men in the UK, hair is lost in a characteristic pattern from the temples and crown (hence the common name male pattern baldness). What starts as a receding hairline and a 'bald spot' at the top of the head progresses, until the two bald areas meet, leaving just a horseshoe pattern of hair above the ears (see figure 3 opposite). Most men get to this stage eventually, but only a few progress beyond it.

The process is usually gradual, rather than sudden, although sometimes it starts and stops. It is rare for a man suffering from genetic hair loss to become completely bald.

In genetic hair loss, the follicles shrink and the diameter of the hairs they produce decreases. Terminal hair is gradually converted into vellus hair, leading to a decrease in the "meaningful hair density" (proportion of non-vellus hair) in the balding area. When the follicles finally stop producing hair, there is a corresponding decrease in the total hair density.

Another feature of genetic hair loss is a shortening of the time the hair spends in the anagen (growing phase), which means that the hair becomes shorter and provides less coverage of the scalp. This also leads to an increase in shedding because the proportion of hairs in the telogen phase must go up as the time spent in anagen goes down.[4] Women may also suffer from genetic hair loss, particularly as they get older. All women produce small amounts of androgens, including DHT. If a woman's hair follicles have an

Figure 3: the Hamilton scale of male genetic hair loss

In men the extent of genetic hair loss is graded using a scale devised by J.B. Hamilton in the 1950s. The diagrams show hair loss on the crown (left) and at the hairline (right).

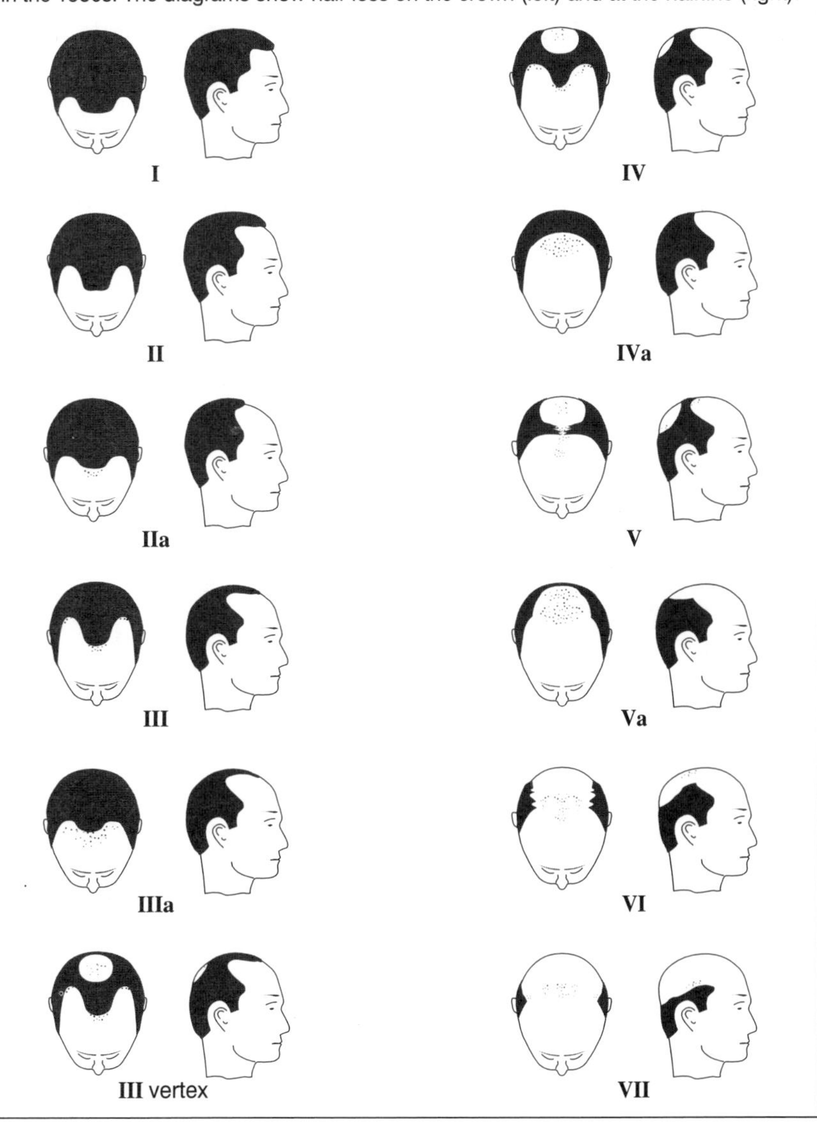

inherited sensitivity to DHT, she may experience hair loss. The condition is thought to affect an estimated 1.4 million women in the UK .

Unlike their male counterparts, these women usually retain their hairline, suffering instead from a diffuse, overall type of thinning (see figure 4 below). Affected women are also likely to complain of widening of hair partings and increased shedding. Although balding women usually have a lower hair density than balding men, the remaining hairs are as thick as those of non-balding women. So women with genetic hair loss usually have much better scalp coverage than balding men do.

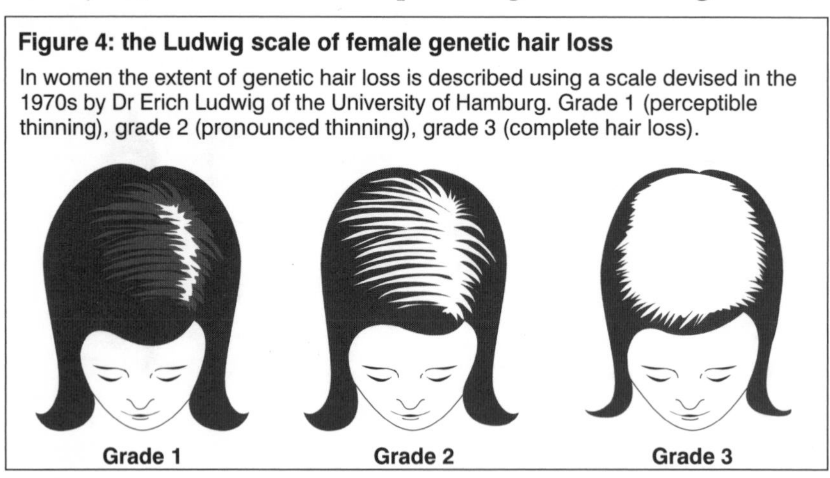

Figure 4: the Ludwig scale of female genetic hair loss

In women the extent of genetic hair loss is described using a scale devised in the 1970s by Dr Erich Ludwig of the University of Hamburg. Grade 1 (perceptible thinning), grade 2 (pronounced thinning), grade 3 (complete hair loss).

Sometimes genetic hair loss in women is accompanied by other symptoms such as acne, or hair growth on the face. Such symptoms usually point to an underlying hormonal disorder such as polycystic ovarian syndrome which, if untreated, can lead to infertility.

Women become more vulnerable to genetic hair loss around the time of the menopause, as their levels of the female sex hormone, oestrogen, fall – exposing them to relatively higher levels of androgens. Hormone replacement therapy (HRT) may shift the hormone balance to either increase or decrease the androgenetic effect, depending on the formulation used. If hair loss runs in your family, make sure your GP or gynaecologist takes this into account if you are considering HRT.

Genetic hair loss can be handed on by either parent, although the strongest influence is on the maternal side. The gene, or genes, responsible for this have not yet been identified and the pattern of inheritance is complex. If hair loss runs in your family, it is likely that you too will be affected, as the following case histories show.

My hair started to go when I was 17. I was prepared, because my father lost his when he was very young and my older brother went bald when he was 26. It does help knowing what to expect. Mike, 31, picture editor.

I've got three older brothers. The eldest didn't start to go bald till he was in his 40's, but the one after him began to lose his hair when he was 19. The one nearest me in age hung onto his hair for a bit longer. My father lost a lot of hair in his early 40's, but then it stopped. He's 75 now and he's got the same hair that he had when he was 50. My mother's two brothers lost some hair, and her father went completely bald from an early age. I knew it would happen to me too. I started to lose my hair when I was 22 and now I've just got bits of hair on either side but I'm completely bald in the middle. Neil, 34, journalist.

But no-one can put a figure on the probability of your losing your hair from a knowledge of your family history

There are also racial differences in the incidence of genetic hair loss. The highest rates are among Caucasians, while Blacks have the second highest incidence. Oriental men and women have the lowest rate, and the condition is unknown among native Americans.

Genetic hair loss is not completely understood, but there is good evidence that it results from an over-sensitivity of the hair follicles to DHT, rather than from raised levels of this hormone in the body. DHT is closely related to another male sex hormone, testosterone, and is produced from it under the influence of an enzyme called 5-alpha reductase.

Testosterone is produced by the testes and also, in far smaller amounts, by the ovaries in women. The first clue to the importance of testosterone in hair loss came from the great Greek physician Hippocrates (who was himself almost completely bald). In 400 BC he wrote "Eunuchs are not subject to gout nor do they become bald". Eunuchs are boys or men whose testicles have been removed or destroyed, and who therefore lack testosterone. Without testosterone there can, of course, be no DHT. If eunuchs are given testosterone, they are as likely to lose their hair as men who have not been castrated.

Both testosterone and DHT are steroid hormones, as are the anabolic steroids that athletes use – illegally – to build muscle and stamina. All steroid hormones act as powerful chemical messengers which regulate biochemical activity within the body cells that they target. Testosterone is responsible for growth of axillary (armpit) and pubic hair at adolescence, as well as male sex drive and aggression. DHT stimulates the growth of facial and body hair. The evidence suggests that it is DHT, not testosterone, which causes the hair follicles to shrink in genetic hair loss.

Women have only about 10 per cent of male levels of either hormone in their follicle cells, which may explain why they suffer a much lower rate of genetic hair loss. However, measuring levels of testosterone, DHT, or 5-alpha reductase in hair follicle tissue does not appear to be a useful predictor of alopecia. There is rarely any evidence of excess levels of testosterone or related hormones in bald men; the belief that baldness makes you more virile than a man with a full head of hair is, unfortunately, without scientific foundation.

Genetic hair loss is irreversible without treatment; this distinguishes the condition from most other forms of alopecia.

It progresses with age, and may be related to the ageing process in some way which is not yet understood. A recent report has uncovered a link between hair loss and smoking[12]. Of 600 male and female patients attending a general surgical outpatient clinic, 35 per cent of the smokers were balding, compared to only 21 per cent of the non-smokers. It is not known whether or how smoking causes baldness. However, smokers do show other signs of ageing such as facial wrinkles and grey hair. This study therefore suggests that baldness may be part of the ageing process, and that smoking is linked in with this in some way.

Treatments which block the action of DHT (so-called anti-androgen therapy) can slow down or stop the hair loss.

Anti-androgen therapy can reverse genetic hair loss in women. In men, the only sure way to reverse baldness is "gender reassignment" – in other words a sex-change operation which involves castration and a change of the hormone profile from male to female. Anti-androgen therapy is discussed in more detail in chapter 8.[8]

Telogen effluvium

Sometimes the hair cycle is interrupted in the anagen phase by a specific event; two to four months later, the affected hairs enter the telogen phase prematurely and are shed all at once.

The clinical name for this rapid diffuse type of hair loss is telogen effluvium. Common triggers for telogen effluvium include prolonged psychological stress, childbirth, surgery, and disorders such as iron deficiency anaemia and/or low iron stores, which may arise from poor diet. The incidence of hair loss after an operation appears to be decreasing, maybe because patients are encouraged to get out of bed earlier than they used to. A fuller list is of possible causes is given in tables

2 and 3. The condition is said to be on the increase, particularly among women as their lives become more stressed, perhaps when they struggle to combine a high-powered job with family responsibilities.[13]

Loss of more than 50 per cent of scalp hair from telogen effluvium is uncommon. If the underlying cause is tackled, the hair should start to regrow two to three months after it has first been shed. Regrowth is usually complete within around 18 months, although the hair may not be as thick as it was before the loss.

TABLE 2

Causes of telogen effluvium

- ◆ Psychological stress (eg divorce, bereavement, road traffic accident)
- ◆ Physical stress (eg surgery)
- ◆ Childbirth
- ◆ Chronic fatigue syndrome (formerly known as myalgic encephalomyelitis or ME)
- ◆ Other disorders such as kidney failure, chronic infection, and cancer
- ◆ Crash dieting, anorexia nervosa
- ◆ Prolonged fever
- ◆ Hormonal disorders (eg underactive thyroid gland)
- ◆ Iron deficiency anaemia
- ◆ Low serum ferritin (iron stores)
- ◆ Common medications (see Table 3)

Telogen effluvium may recur, and if the cause is not treated, the hair loss may persist for a long time.

Anagen effluvium

Hair loss is a frequent side effect of cancer chemotherapy, because anti-cancer drugs target any rapidly dividing cells in the body. This means they damage not only cancer cells but also healthy dividing cells such as those in the matrix of the hair follicle, during the anagen phase. The resulting hair loss,

TABLE 3

Drugs which may lead to hair loss as a side effect*

◆ Withdrawal from oral contraceptives◆ Physical stress (eg surgery)

◆ Anticoagulants: heparin, warfarin

◆ Antidepressants: imipramine (Tofranil), desipramine (Pertofran), fluoxetine (Prozac) and lithium (used for manic depression)

◆ Drugs used in the treatment of high blood pressure eg beta blockers: propanolol (Inderal), metoprolol (Lopresor, Betaloc), nadolol (Corgard) and angiotensin converting enzyme (ACE)

◆ Inhibitors: captopril (Capoten, Acepril), enalapril (Innovace)

◆ Antithyroid medications: propylthiouracil

◆ Treatment for Parkinson's disease: laevodopa (Brocadopa, Larodopa) nicotinic acid (used to lower cholesterol)

*(generic names listed, trade names in brackets)

which is known as anagen effluvium, is characterised by a reduction in the growth rate of the hair and by thinning and breakage of the hair shafts. Typically a patchy hair loss sets in two to four weeks after the start of treatment. Up to 90 per cent of scalp hair may be lost.

Intravenous chemotherapy leads to more hair loss than oral anti-cancer drugs. The drugs most often associated with anagen effluvium are doxorubicin, vincristine and methotrexate, which are used to treat many kinds of cancer, and cyclophosphamide, used mainly in the treatment of Hodgkin's disease and leukemia.

However, hair loss can be prevented or minimised by cooling the scalp. For more details, see chapter 5.

Hair that is lost following cancer chemotherapy usually regrows three to six months after it first falls out – even if the treatment is still going on. It may well be thicker than before chemotherapy when it does come back.[6]

Alopecia areata

Sudden loss of hair in oval patches from the scalp is known as alopecia areata. It affects two per cent of the population at some time in their life. In alopecia areata, the bald patches are surrounded by characteristic broken, tapered hairs, known as "exclamation mark" hairs. When all the hair on the scalp is lost, the condition is known as alopecia totalis. Other hair bearing areas of the body may be affected by alopecia areata; in alopecia totalis eyelashes and eyebrows are also lost, and in alopecia universalis, all the body hair is lost too.

Most of those affected by alopecia areata are children and young adults; only 25 per cent of sufferers are over 40.

There is often a family history of the disease, and it may occur alongside Down syndrome, Addison's disease, or vitiligo (a disorder in which unpigmented pale patches appear on the skin.)

Often other associated symptoms such as pitting of the nails occur along with the hair loss.

I began to lose my hair when I was 13. The hairdresser noticed a small bald patch about the size of a ten pence piece on the side of my head. Kids at school thought I must have cancer. By the time I was 16, I was wearing a wig. Now I have no hair, eyelashes or eyebrows – nothing. The doctors say that the longer it goes on, the less likely it is to come back. Eilidh, 27, clerical officer.

Alopecia areata is thought to be an autoimmune disease. In autoimmune disease, the immune system appears to lose the ability to distinguish between "self" and "not self". Instead of restricting itself to attacking foreign invaders, such as bacterial or viral infections, it also turns on the body's own tissues and starts to destroy them. Other autoimmune diseases include rheumatoid arthritis, systemic lupus erythematosus (SLE) and possibly multiple sclerosis.

Alopecia areata is a very unpredictable condition. There is a ten per cent chance that all the hair will regrow spontaneously, even after many years. The hair often comes back during pregnancy, probably because pregnancy causes changes in the immune system. Treatment with steroids or minoxidil (see chapter 8) may help regrowth. The outlook is less hopeful in alopecia totalis, and alopecia universalis, although there is a great deal of research going on into the condition.[5, 14]

Traumatic alopecia

Patchy hair loss and twisted broken off hair may be caused by treating the hair and scalp badly. In friction alopecia, tightly fitting hats and wigs lead to hair loss. Certain hairdressing practices lead to traction alopecia by pulling too tightly on the hair. Tightly wound hair curlers, tight hair braiding, and hot comb treatment used to straighten curly hair are the main causes of traction alopecia. Occasionally a perm will damage the scalp and lead to hair loss. Generally, these forms of traumatic alopecia resolve once the cause is identified and remedied.

In trichotillomania, people inflict hair loss on themselves by pulling out their own hair. The disorder is fairly common in children and especially in young women between the ages of 16 and 20. If it persists into adult life, it may be symptomatic of a serious underlying psychological disorder which is best treated by psychotherapy or medication.

When I was 15 or 16, I began to pull out my hair. No-one took it that seriously because I came from a happy family. We just thought it was a bad habit I had. Many years later it turned out that the I had been suffering from a mild form of manic depression. This got worse a couple of years ago, but now I'm taking medication, and it's under control. But they say my hair won't grow back now. I'll probably be buried in my beautiful real hair wig. Ann, 45, business consultant

Scalp infection

Scalp infections can lead to hair loss. Fungal infections such as tinea capitis (scalp ringworm) are commoner in children than in adults and cause itchy patches of baldness. Folliculitis is a bacterial scalp infection which causes pustules and diffuse alopecia. The other, less common, bacterial infection is pyoderma which leads to a red, scaly scalp and either patchy or diffuse hair loss.

Hair loss is also seen in systemic lupus erythematosus, a chronic inflammatory disease which occurs mainly in women of child-bearing age. It can give rise to scaling, redness and broken off hairs. Psoriasis, a chronic skin disease characterised by thick, red inflamed patches all over the body may also be associated with hair loss.

But are you really losing your hair?

Finally, there is a rare psychological disorder called dysmorphophobia in which patients whose hair is perfectly normal believe they have alopecia. These patients may be suffering from unresolved anxiety, relationship difficulties and/or depressive illness and are displacing their distress onto their hair.

Treating people with dysmorphophobia may take longer than helping patients with genuine alopecia and it can be difficult to persuade them to accept psychiatric help.

Chapter 3

How hair loss affects you

Although hair loss has no effect on your physical health, it may well have a huge impact on your psychological well being. A full head of hair is associated with youth and sexual attractiveness in both men and women. And in an increasingly image-conscious society first impressions are all-important. Losing your hair can drastically alter the way you look, and so deliver a crushing blow to your self-esteem. This, in turn, may cause social withdrawal, lack of confidence in social and sexual situations, and feelings of discomfort and self-consciousness in public. At its worst, distress over hair loss can result in clinical depression, despair and suicide.

Yet some people appear to take hair loss in their stride.

The Australian TV critic Clive James calls them "own-up baldies". You won't find these people shelling out for a hair transplant, expensive scalp lotions or a wig. Nor will they attempt to comb their existing hair over their bald patch, or cover it with a hat. Instead they might even hurry the natural course of the balding process by shaving their heads completely.

Famous own-up baldies include Clive James himself, TV presenter Clive Anderson, movie stars Sean Connery and Bruce Willis, and actor Ross Kemp (Grant Mitchell in East Enders).

But being rich and famous doesn't always make people feel good about being bald. Pop star Elton John hid his baldness with a cap for many years before opting for a hair transplant. Cricketer Graham Gooch has a hair weave (and appeared on advertisements for the clinic who carried out the treatment).

There is no way of predicting how people will react to hair loss, but it seems to hit women, and men who go bald early, particularly hard. The reasons are obvious; balding among older men is commonplace – but women and young men who lose their hair really do stand out from the crowd. Sudden hair loss, which is the hallmark of telogen effluvium and alopecia areata, is particularly upsetting. Some cancer patients will even refuse chemotherapy because they just cannot cope with the prospect of losing their hair as a result.

All in the mind?

Hair loss might be easier to accept if it could be proved that being bald does not stop you getting on in life. After all, as we have just seen, there are many successful people who have lost, or are losing, their hair. But there is some evidence that baldness can have a negative impact on the way people react to you.

The president of the United States has a full head of hair. There has not been a bald president within living memory. And there is a lower proportion of bald men in Congress than in the general US population. A recent episode of the cartoon show *The Simpsons* hinted at what Americans really think of bald men. Hero Homer Simpson, normally seen with just two remaining strands of hair on an otherwise bald pate, paid out $1000 for a hair loss lotion (whose name was a sly anagram of the only licensed over-the-counter drug for baldness – of which more in chapter 8). When Homer grew back, overnight, the long flowing locks he'd had in his teens, he was immediately promoted to the executive board of his company. But as soon as his hair fell out again, Homer was back on the production line.

The British seem to be equally prejudiced. Grant and Phil Mitchell may be sex symbols in the television soap opera *East*

Enders, but when it comes to political power, you need hair. We have not had a bald prime minister since Sir Winston Churchill. When the Labour Party leader Tony Blair "came out" recently about his own thinning locks, after a media fuss over an apparent change in his hairstyle, *The Times* was quick to seize on this important political trend. But in France, bald political leaders are the rule rather than the exception – from presidents Charles de Gaulle and François Mitterrand to the present prime minister Alain Juppé.

Are these trends just coincidence? Or could baldness really be a barrier to high political office (or success in other walks of life)? A team of US psychologists set up a study to discover the answer. They created two different "election leaflets" for models with moderate to severe hair loss posing as political candidates. One leaflet had a photo of the model in his natural state, while the other showed him fitted with a hairpiece. Both leaflets contained information about the "candidate's" background and beliefs. Volunteer judges admitted the models looked younger with the hairpiece. But they did not rate them as being any more masculine, attractive, dynamic or pleasant with the hairpiece than in their natural balding state.[1]

This experiment might suggest that hair loss really does not affect people's impressions of you. But, remember, there was written information available about the "candidate" which may have influenced the volunteers' opinions. Thomas Cash of Old Dominion University, Norfolk, Virginia, specialises in the psychology of baldness and body image and has carried out experiments which may better reflect those vital first impressions. He photographed 18 pairs of volunteers who were similar in age and appearance. The only difference was that one in the pair was bald, and the other was not. Then he showed the pictures to volunteers and asked for their reactions.

Overall the volunteers rated the balding partner of each pair as being less attractive, less successful, and less assertive than the non-balding partner. What was particularly striking was the tendency to overestimate the age of the balding men and underestimate the age of the men with hair. On average, the volunteers thought the balding men were up to 3 years older than they actually were, while the non-balding men were seen as around 2 years younger than their real age.

There was some good news for the bald men though;on the whole, they were not seen as being less intelligent than their hairy counterparts. And there were intriguing sex differences in the volunteers' reactions. While young women, unfortunately, gave the thumbs down to the bald young men, more mature women actually preferred them – perhaps because they seemed more mature than men with a good head of hair.[6]

Of course, these experiments have their limitations.

Seeing a photo of someone for the first time is no substitute for meeting them in the flesh, talking to them, and getting to know them. People have more to offer than their hair – or lack of it!

A problem of self image

We simply do not know how the majority of people feel about losing their hair, because most do not ask for help. This could be because they are quite happy to be bald, or that they are upset about their hair loss but feel there is no help available. There have been some surveys of patients in hair clinics which show that they do suffer loss of self esteem and related psychological symptoms because of their hair loss.[2, 3, 5]

However, this data is not very revealing because these people are really a self-selected group – they must be distressed by their baldness to go to a clinic in the first place.

Pamela Wells, a psychologist at Goldsmith's College London,

recently reported an important study of how concerned the average person might be over his or her hair loss. She and her team approached 182 men drawn from the local area, with occupations ranging from doctor to postman, and asked them to fill in a personality questionnaire. None of the volunteers knew the survey was about baldness, but the psychologists secretly recorded their degree of hair loss.

The results showed that hair loss does produce a degree of low self esteem, depression and introversion. The negative effects were, as might have been expected, more pronounced in younger men.[1]

What is not known from this study, is whether hair loss actually produces psychological distress, or alternatively, whether baldness results – in some unknown way – from low self-esteem. Dr Wells comments that the level of psychological suffering she uncovered was surprising, and worthy of further study. The experience of one of her subjects speaks for itself:

I just felt incredibly ugly – a bit of a freak. It just seemed so unfair and I was desperately unhappy. It wasn't long before my girlfriend split with me. I seriously wanted to kill myself and was just so unbelievably depressed . . . I felt I had nothing to look forward to. I think it was probably worse for me because I had always prided myself on my looks – I think my looks were my major asset. I still think I'm pretty good looking when I wear a hat . . . as you know, I never go anywhere without my hat on. I know everyone knows I'm bald but I still think I look better with my hat on – only two people have ever seen me with my hat off in the past three years . . . you know it's no coincidence that my present job is as a chef just so that I can wear a hat . . .

Two years on (at age 23 he had attempted suicide):

I wouldn't say I'm any longer suicidal but I do still get really depressed about it . . . I haven't had a girlfriend now for nearly two years. I have much less confidence than I used to have and I don't go out nearly as much. In a way, I'm looking forward to getting older – being bald won't be so bad then. (Reproduced with the kind permission of the British Journal of Psychology.)

Other men manage to take hair loss in their stride.

People make comments all the time, but I just ignore them.

If you're bald, people tend to think you're older and more experienced than you are. You get taken more seriously. I'd say the only drawback is in the summer, when I always seem to end up with a sunburned head.

I never considered a transplant, and I would never, ever wear a wig. My advice to anyone losing their hair is – if it's going to go, it will. You've just got to learn to live with it. Mike, 31, picture editor.

I was very annoyed when I first started losing my hair. I didn't want it to happen. I forked out for laser treatment, massage, and I even tried Regaine® for a while in the first two or three years. Then I decided to stop wasting my time. People will occasionally make a comment, but I try to get in first. I work for a women's magazine and the place is full of beautiful people. Occasionally I'll feel less than attractive in comparison, but I try to make a feature of something else instead of bothering about my lack of hair.

But if I could have my hair back, I would. I even have hair in my dreams. My advice to anyone worried about hair loss is that if it's going to happen you have to learn to live with it.

Personally, I don't think there's an alternative to going bald. It has more joke value if you try to hide it. It's never convincing. I would rather people laughed at me because I was losing my hair than if I tried to cover up the fact. Neil, 34, journalist.

Women suffer more

If men find baldness upsetting, women find it more so. Hardly surprising, as there is more pressure on women to look attractive than there is on men. Thomas Cash did a special study of the psychological impact of genetic hair loss on women. He talked to 96 women and 60 men with the condition, and compared their responses with those of 56 women with other – less visible – skin complaints. In general, women found hair loss more of a stress than the men did; it did more harm to their body image and self-esteem and

TABLE 4

The top ten complaints of women with hair loss and their percentage frequency compared to the results in men

	Women	Men
Wish that I had more hair	**98**	**90**
Think about my hair loss	**97**	**93**
Try to figure out if I am losing more hair (by inspecting my head, my brush, my sink)	**95**	**87**
Feel frustrated or helpless about my hair loss	**93**	**88**
Spend time looking at my hair/head in the mirror	**92**	**92**
Worry about my looks	**92**	**85**
Feel self-conscious about my looks	**92**	**78**
Have negative thoughts about my hair/head	**91**	**85**
Worry about whether others will notice my hair loss	**90**	**82**
Worry about how much hair I am going to lose	**89**	**93**

produced more social anxiety. Twice as many women as men described themselves as either "very" or "extremely" upset by their hair loss.[7]

A particularly interesting observation was that patients' distress was in proportion to the amount of hair loss they thought they had. This did not always match the assessment of the dermatologist or hair stylist.

It is very rare for someone upset about hair loss to be referred to a psychologist or psychiatrist. In fact, such people could be helped by counselling or therapy directed at improving their body image.[4]

But it is possible to work through the distress without professional help. Here, in a poem, one woman describes how she came to terms with hair loss over a period of several years.

GOING BACK TO MY ROOTS

When it began at first
All I did was cry
I asked myself.
Why me? Oh why?

What had I done wrong?
Was I really that bad?
To cause all this upset
To my Mum and Dad

They tried to console me
But it did no good
I just wasn't listening
They tried all they could

So it wasn't just me
Who was suffering this
It hurt those who love me
That's one thing I don't miss

I've put it behind me
I'm looking ahead
I'm no longer crying
I'm laughing instead

There's nothing to call me
That's not already been said
And all this because
There's not a hair on my head

That's right – I'm a baldie
So now do you see
But listen dear reader
The last laugh's on me

I don't spend my money
On all that hair stuff
I use Fairy Liquid
For me that's enough

I don't have bad hair days
My roots don't show through
I wouldn't swap places
With someone like you

I've got a few hairdos
From which I can pick
Long ones and short one
Bet I'm making you sick

If I fancy a change
I just pick up a book
And choose a new style
To achieve that new look

It took a long time
But I'm settled at last
The years of despair
Are all in the past

Now I'm coping with this
I would say it's a plus
I get up in the morning
Hey presto – no fuss

No tangles no cow licks
I just put my hair on
Put on my eyelashes
Ten minutes and I'm gone

So now that I'm happy
And on the right track
I no longer know
If I want my hair back

I'm mousey brown one day
The next I'm a blonde
If you want my opinion
You're all getting conned

All these shampoos on telly
Are cashing in big
Buy a bottle of Fairy
And put the squeak on your wig

So you'll not see me looking
At the hair dyes in Boots
Take a tip from me reader
And go back to your roots!

Eilidh Fraser

Chapter 4

Self help for hair

So maybe you are suffering from some degree of hair loss. Don't panic. Before you start thinking about wigs, transplants and hair restoring lotions (which will be discussed in later chapters), why not look first at how to make the most of the hair you still have – and how to stop losing even more?

The way you and your hairdresser look after your hair, plus your general lifestyle, can have a big impact on hair loss problems. It could be time for a complete re-think of your hair care routine.

Handling your hair

Most people tend to be too rough with their hair. Start treating it with a bit more respect. First check out your combs and brushes. If your hair is thinning, it is generally better to use a comb rather than a brush, because it is harder to apply excessive force with a comb. Vigorous brushing weakens the hair and may well pull it out if done over a period of time. Avoid any sharp spikes which could damage the scalp. This means steering clear of metal and natural bristle. The best combs and brushes have widely spaced blunt teeth, and are made of vulcanite (hard rubber).

Remember that traction alopecia is caused by anything that pulls on your hair, or causes excessive friction between the scalp and the hair. For instance, tightly-fitting hats and caps may cover balding patches, but can actually increase hair loss by causing friction between the hair and the scalp. The same goes for pony tails, and tight braids. When you pull on hair, it does extend – but only to a certain limit. Beyond this it just breaks off. If you do wear a pony tail, secure it with a fabric band. Elastic bands cut into the hair shaft, and when you remove it some hair usually comes away with it. Shampooing cleans the hair and the scalp. People sometimes worry that frequent shampooing makes hair fall out more. It doesn't – if you shampoo it properly. Athletes, and other people who wash their hair frequently, suffer no more hair loss than people who wash their hair less often. You can wash your hair every day if you like. In fact, if your hair is thinning, the more often you wash, the thicker and fluffier it will look. When hair is dirty it tends to stick together, which makes it look thinner.

Effective shampooing starts with selecting the right shampoo for your hair. This can be tricky, as there are hundreds of different products on the market. Beware of hairdressers who tell you that only expensive salon products will do. Supermarket and high street chemists' shampoos can be equally effective, at only a fraction of the cost – but it's worth finding one that suits your hair type. Instead of worrying about the hair you're losing, think for a moment about what is left.

Is it dry or greasy? Fine or thick? And has it been damaged in any way – by too much sun, perhaps, or chemical treatments such as colouring or perming?

All shampoos contain detergent. Like washing-up liquid, or soap powder, they lock onto grease and gently lift it from the surface it's sticking to (hair, in the case of shampoo) and wash it away in the rinsing water. Soap was the original detergent but it has been replaced in most modern shampoos by soapless detergents, derived from petroleum, such as sodium lauryl sulphate.

A good shampoo creates plenty of lather which spreads the detergent easily over the hair. Otherwise you have to rub it in too hard which creates unnecessary friction. And this, of course, weakens the hair. At the same time, the shampoo must wet the hair properly so that it comes into contact with the dirt.

During shampooing, the hair will absorb up to 30 per cent of its own weight of water, if wetting is effective.

The amount of detergent in your shampoo is important and should be matched carefully to your hair type. The higher the percentage of detergent, the more your hair will be "degreased" after shampooing. If you have oily hair, you could go for a shampoo containing up to 50 per cent detergent. But people with dry hair need a shampoo with, say, 10-20 per cent detergent to stop the natural sebum being washed out of their hair and leaving it in a degreased condition which may be more vulnerable to breakage.

Frequent wash shampoos also have a low proportion of detergent and should be used if you like to shampoo daily, even if your hair is oily. Otherwise detergent will strip your hair of its natural oils.

Some shampoos have added vegetable oils such as coconut, almond and olive or waxes like lanolin and jojoba, which resemble sebum. These are good if you have dry hair, as they counteract the degreasing effect of the detergent. They also have a conditioning effect, leaving the hair smoother and easier to comb. And the easier it is to pull a comb or brush through your hair, the less likely it is to break off.

You may also find a protein-based shampoo useful. These products do not contain protein as such and so cannot actually "feed" the hair. Instead, they contain the constituents of proteins, which are amino acids and peptides. These are able to cling to the surface of the hair cuticle, making it smooth, or penetrate the interior of the shaft and make chemical linkages which temporarily "repair" damaged hair.

Acid balanced shampoos may help restore the hair to its natural slightly acidic condition after chemical treatments, and can smooth down the cuticle – making hair easier to comb through. They contain natural organic acids, such as citric acid. Lemons contain citric acid, so this is the basis of the lemon or vinegar rinse to make hair shiny after shampooing. Some shampoos contain ingredients such as menthol or silicone which are specifically meant to prevent hair loss.

While there is no sound medical evidence that these stop hair falling out, or restore hair to bald patches, it is worth trying them out to see if they improve the state of your own hair. Menthol is supposed to increase the blood supply to the hair roots, while silicone coats the hair cuticles and makes it look thicker. The Body Shop's *Ice Blue* shampoo contains menthol, or you could try *Menthol Shampoo* and *Menthol Lotion* from the Scalp and Hair Clinic (contact details at the end of chapter 5).

And it's not just the shampoo you select that affects the state of your hair – it's the way you use it. Do not apply shampoo to dry hair; wet it first. And dilute your shampoo – one teaspoon in an eggcup of warm water is about right – before you apply it to your hair. Most of us don't pay enough attention to rinsing our hair after shampooing. Take a tip from hairdressers. They are taught to use 20 litres of warm water (just above body temperature) to rinse out a shampoo. Use less and you risk scalp irritation, which may well aggravate any tendency to hair loss.

While your hair is wet, you do need to take more care in the way you handle it. Wet hair extends more than dry hair - that's why hairdressers style and perm it when wet because it is easier to manipulate. But it is also more prone to over-stretching, and breaking, when it is wet. So you need to be even gentler when you are combing it through. Be very patient when you are removing tangles. Get to work on them with a wide-toothed comb before rinsing out your conditioner. Start at the ends and gently work up to the roots. Do not rinse until you can comb right through your hair from the roots to the ends.

Conditioner is essential, by the way, every time you shampoo. It smooths down the cells in the cuticles of the hair and prevents tangling. Once these cells lie flat, they reflect more light making your hair look shiny and healthy (which, of course, distracts attention from a balding scalp). Conditioners also moisturise the hair, and may coat the shaft giving extra body. As with shampoo, you may need to shop around to find the best conditioner for your hair. You may want to add a "volumising" styling aid such as a spray, mousse or gel before drying if the conditioner does not provide enough body on its own.

Excessive heat from a hairdryer, a hot comb, or rollers can make your hair break through a form of traction alopecia. Letting your hair dry naturally causes least damage but gives you no opportunity for styling. And without styling, you are missing out on an opportunity to make your hair look thicker and more abundant.

However the hair is dried you are likely to use a towel to get rid of excess wetness. Be gentle and blot away the water rather than rubbing vigorously with a towel. And if you then use a hairdryer, only use maximum heat when your hair is still wet.

Reduce the heat as your hair dries. It is best to leave it very slightly damp if you can. Using a hairdryer on nearly dry hair is risky – it may overdry the hair, making it weak and brittle. If you use rollers or a heat comb, be really gentle; pulling too hard may lead to traction alopecia.

If ordinary shampoos and conditioners still expose your hair loss, you might want to consider using special products to make more of your hair. There are many thickening sprays which coat the hair with polymer, for instance. Try *Thicker Fuller Hair* or *Maximizer* from Philip Kingsley (contact details at the end of chapter 5).[5]

There are also "fogging" products – powder sprays which colour your scalp the same shade as your hair. They have the effect of minimising the contrast between your hair and any bald patches. They will cost you around £15 for a few months' supply.

Try *Mane* or *Top Secret*. There is more about hair care products for people with thinning hair in chapter 9.[1,2]

You and your hairdresser

If you are worried about hair loss, now is the time to review your relationship with your hairdresser and take a long cool look at what he or she has to offer. Ideally, you'll sit down together and take time to talk about things like your lifestyle, hair type, face and head shape, your hair's growing pattern and, of course, the reason why you're losing your hair. The basis of good hairdressing is a decent cut. And it's perhaps worth having it done more often if your hair is thinning; once every six to eight weeks is ideal. The type of cut you have depends on your hair but in general, the rule is the shorter the better. Don't be tempted to grow the rest of your hair long (or, men, facial hair where you didn't have it before – the general effect is ageing). Long hair, with a bald or thinning patch, only draws people's attention to your hair.

Short hair minimises the contrast between the thinning and hair-bearing area. Get your hairdresser to thin it out so it looks the same all over.

A layered hair cut is usually a good option to create bulk in your remaining hair. However, women with longer hair may find it better to keep it all one length to maximise body and volume.

But anything 'bouffant' (remember Tony Blair) will only emphasise lack of hair elsewhere. A flat hairstyle is generally more flattering.

As far as an individual style is concerned, it really depends upon the shape of your face and head and where your hair is thinning. Women with thinning hair should avoid a central parting, for example. Don't discount a perm to add fullness and texture; it works for men and women alike, but make sure you use a reputable hairdresser because perming lotion can damage your hair[3, 6].

Even colouring can help disguise hair loss. Ask your hairdresser to tint your hair lighter, for instance. This will lessen the contrast between your hair and bald patches on your scalp. It may also give a useful illusion of depth and texture.

Colour rinses (which wash out after shampooing) decrease the shininess of bald scalp, making it look less obvious. And many colouring agents make the hair shaft swell, and so make the remaining hair look thicker.

Men have a strange attitude towards colouring their hair.

According to trichologist Philip Kingsley, most wait until they are completely grey, panic, and then go for a progressive hair dye. This is supposed to restore the hair colour gradually, but rarely looks natural. It is far better to start tinting when the hair colour starts to fade, and try semi-permanent dyes which are aimed at women (sometimes you can find them discreetly packaged for men), or ask your hairdresser for advice on a permanent colour.

Apart from styling, perming, and colouring, there are also some treatments which your hairdresser can give which may improve the condition of your hair. Massage, for example, increases the blood supply to the hair follicles, and when done on a regular basis may delay hair loss. A well-trained hairdresser or trichologist should use a number of massage techniques; and at least you should find the process relaxing, which in turn might make you feel better about your hair loss, even if it continues to fall out (for more about relaxation and hair loss see chapter 9). It is also good to massage your own scalp by kneading it gently, at least once a week, after applying a good scalp lotion. This will exercise the scalp muscles, and should help keep your follicles in good condition.

Heat treatment, using hot towels, steam or infra-red lamps has a similar effect in encouraging an increase in the blood supply to the scalp. You might consider high frequency electrical treatment (best from a qualified trichologist after correct diagnosis of your hair problem); this too increases blood flow to the hair follicles. The high frequency equipment consists of a box plugged into mains electricity. This is connected to a glass device in the shape of a comb or bulb massager which the hairdresser applies to the scalp. The electric current you receive is tiny, so there is no danger of electric shock. However, the direction of the current changes many times per second and this has a heating effect which, in turn, increases the blood supply to the scalp.

Diet and lifestyle

Poor nutrition, in general, can certainly lead to hair loss. Any nutrients in short supply will be diverted from the scalp towards areas of the body which need them more. People who go on crash diets, or suddenly become vegetarian often find that their hair falls out as a result. So make sure you follow a sensible low-fat diet high in fruit and vegetables, and with sufficient protein and carbohydrate.[4]

The protein component of your diet is especially important; hair is made of a protein called keratin. Protein in the diet is broken down by enzymes in the digestive system into basic components called amino acids. These are then transported by the blood to all the tissues of the body, where they're used to build up the proteins that the body needs – in the case of the hair follicles, the protein is keratin.

If you are not a vegetarian, good protein sources in your diet would include fish and chicken. If you don't eat meat, you should plan your diet carefully to combine different protein sources. The reason is that while animal protein contains all the amino acids the body needs, plant proteins do not. Plant foods can be divided into three groups depending on their amino acid composition; grains, legumes (peas and beans), and nuts and seeds. If you combine foods from at least two of these groups at a meal, you will be getting your full quota of amino acids. Try combinations such as beans on toast, peanut butter sandwiches, and ethnic dishes such as vegetarian chilli and rice, or lentil or pea curry with Indian breads.

If you are not getting sufficient vitamins and minerals, your hair could be affected. Vitamins B, C and E are particularly important for the health of your hair. Among the B vitamins, B12 – which may be lacking in vegan diets – folic acid, and biotin appear to affect hair growth the most. Good sources of B vitamins include soya beans, dairy products, fish, eggs and liver. Vitamin C is found in many fresh fruits and vegetables, and particularly in citrus fruits such as oranges and lemons. Lack of vitamin E leads to thinning fur in animals; you will find vitamin E in dairy products, nuts and seeds, and vegetable oils.

Trace amounts of minerals are also necessary for the hair.

Lack of iron and zinc, in particular, are suspected to play a role in hair loss. Red meat and leafy vegetables like spinach are high in iron. Zinc is found in shellfish, peas and beans. Recent research strongly suggests that the total amount of iron stored in the body may be more important than the level of iron in the red blood cells where the health of the hair is concerned. Iron stores are estimated by measuring serum ferritin (ferritin is a protein which stores iron). Haemoglobin levels are a measure of the amount of iron in your blood cells. Low levels suggest iron deficiency anaemia, a condition which is fairly common among vegetarians, women who have heavy periods, and anyone with a generally poor diet. However, many women with a hair loss problem have low serum ferritin, even though their haemoglobin is normal. Women are far more prone to low ferritin than men. Maybe the years of menstruation (uninterrupted, in these days of effective contraception, by one pregnancy after another) draw on their iron stores as the body attempts to keep up adequate levels of haemoglobin. Women with a persistent hair loss problem could ask their doctor to check their serum ferritin as well as their haemoglobin levels.

If you want to put all this together and eat for the optimum health of your hair, you could try Philip Kingsley's *Seven Day Hair Vitality Diet* (details at the end of this chapter).

Should you take supplements? As far as protein is concerned, this should always come from your diet. Supplements of individual amino acids are not usually a good idea. However, vegetarians and vegans might want to look at blue green algae products such as Chlorella and Spirulina. Like animal proteins, these contain all the amino acids you need. They come as a powder which you can sprinkle into soups and other dishes. Or you can take them in tablet form. While there's no firm evidence that blue green algae can really help with hair loss, they won't do you any harm if you follow the instructions on the packet.

And if you find it hard to improve the protein content of your diet any other way, they may be worth a try.

As far as vitamins are concerned, if you are getting five (or more) helpings of fresh fruit and vegetables a day (this includes juices and tinned – but not dry or pickled – products) you should not be deficient in any of them. At least, that's the official view. However, some nutritionists think that the recommended daily allowances are too low. If you decide to try a supplement, it is best to take a B complex with all the vitamins rather than just B12, folic acid or biotin. A gram of vitamin C a day will do you no harm: if you take more you may get diarrhoea and will certainly be wasting your money. Check with your doctor before taking vitamin E if you are on anti-coagulants.

Iron supplements should never be taken without professional advice or on prescription, but zinc (as zinc citrate or zinc gluconate) can be bought from a chemist's or health food shop. Zinc can interfere with the action of other nutrients in the body; it is best not to take more than 30-50 mg a day. Zinc tablets are best taken alone, last thing at night.

NutriHair®, which has been developed by Hugh Rushton – who has done much of the research into female hair loss and low ferritin – contains iron along with lysine, vitamin B12 and vitamin C. There is evidence that deficiency of lysine, an amino acid, may also contribute to chronic telogen effluvium in women. NutriHair® is available from Nature's Best by mail order. It will take up to 16 weeks before you notice a reduction in hair shedding on NutriHair®; if there has been no improvement after nine months, your hair loss is due to some other cause and you should seek further advice.

Apart from feeding your body properly, there are maybe some other improvements you could make to your lifestyle. Avoid stress wherever possible. Regular exercise, counselling, massage and relaxation techniques are all effective. When you are stressed, the muscles in your scalp tense up, restricting the flow of blood to the hair follicles. Dress as well as you can afford and look after your skin to make sure people don't find your bald spot the most interesting thing about your appearance.

Further reading

Hair: An owner's Handbook, Philip Kingsley, Aurum, £12.95

Chapter 5

Remedies for hair loss

You may have reached the point where you want professional help with a hair problem. Your reason probably falls into one of the following categories:

- ❑ the amount of hair you have lost or are losing is not acceptable to you;
- ❑ you have had previous treatment for hair loss which has not worked;
- ❑ you are concerned about future hair loss because you need chemotherapy for cancer

Where to seek help for hair loss

To get advice and treatment for hair loss you should start with either your GP or a with professionally qualified trichologist. Whether you choose to approach your doctor depends on several factors. Until recently, genetic hair loss in men has been seen as a natural process. Most doctors are unlikely to be sympathetic or helpful to balding male patients. However, there are signs that the medical profession is beginning to wake up to the fact that genetic hair loss can lead to a significant decrease in quality of life, especially for younger men. If you are lucky enough to have an enlightened GP you may at least get some useful advice.

Genetic hair loss in women, on the other hand, is usually seen as being pathological. With this, and other forms of hair loss, such as alopecia areata, the GP should either treat you himself or refer you to a dermatologist at the hospital.

A dermatologist is a doctor specialising in the diagnosis and treatment of skin problems. This includes hair loss, but in practice only a handful of dermatologists in the UK have much experience or knowledge of hair problems. The best, like Dr David Fenton of the Hair Research Clinic at St Thomas's Hospital in London, have carried out extensive research into the causes of hair loss and are currently investigating several new treatments. But many dermatologists will tell you that there is nothing they can do to help.

The other option is to consult a trichologist – especially if you are sure your hair loss is not a sign of a serious underlying disorder which needs medical treatment. A trichologist is a hair specialist whose training covers both cosmetic and medical aspects of the subject. Some trichologists are also trained hairdressers, but they are not medically qualified in the sense that a doctor or nurse is. Anyone can set up as a trichologist, but the Institute of Trichologists keeps a register of people who are properly qualified. Look for the letters AIT (Associate), MIT (Member), or FIT (Fellow) when you are choosing a trichologist. The Institute can provide you with a list of registered trichologists in your area (details are given below).

An ethical trichologist will give you a realistic assessment of your situation and what can be done about it. Be prepared for this. You may not like what they have to say. For instance, they may be fairly pessimistic about the chances of slowing your hair loss, or the likelihood of it regrowing.

If you are very depressed by your hair loss, you may be tempted instead by one of the many clinics which seem to offer a more optimistic outlook. They advertise extensively in newspapers and in Yellow Pages. Some are perfectly genuine, others are just after your money. If you want to try a clinic, do ask the Institute of Trichologists for advice first. Details of some well-established clinics with a good reputation are also given below.

Before you embark on treatment that could be expensive (and has no guarantee of success) it is worth asking yourself just why your hair loss bothers you so much. No-one likes going bald, but many people just accept it (see chapter 3). Obviously if hair loss is a symptom of a serious underlying medical condition then you must get treatment. But could your dissatisfaction with your hair be masking another problem – such as fear of ageing, depression, or a lack of confidence? If there is a grain of truth in this, it might be worth talking things over with a counsellor before tackling your hair loss. This also applies if you have tried many hair loss treatments and found them all unsatisfactory.

Finally, if you are about to undergo cancer chemotherapy there is a strong possibility that you will lose much, if not all, of your hair (see chapter 2). However, this can be prevented by cooling the scalp while the drug is being administered (the treatment is discussed in more detail below).

The oncologist (cancer specialist) will advise whether this is available at the hospital and whether it is applicable in your particular case.

Investigating and diagnosing hair loss

Although there are many different causes of hair loss, in the majority of cases diagnosis should be fairly straightforward.

Most balding men are suffering from genetic hair loss. Around 90 per cent of women complaining of hair loss have either chronic telogen effluvium, or genetic hair loss.

A doctor or trichologist can tell immediately if a man has genetic hair loss. The characteristic pattern of a receding hairline and a thinning crown speaks for itself, especially if the patient is over 25. A family history of hair loss clinches the diagnosis and no further investigation is needed. In all other cases, a complete medical history should be taken. Recent stresses, both physical and psychological, may be useful pointers to telogen effluvium. Other symptoms, such as fatigue or dry skin, indicate a possible thyroid problem or another underlying illness.

The doctor should also ask about your hair care routine, in case you have traumatic alopecia, and about any drugs you are taking such as oral contraceptives or prescription medicines.

Many drugs can cause hair loss as a side effect (see table 3).

A physical examination might also be useful. This should include the whole skin surface – not just your scalp. The doctor will look at your hair loss pattern (remember, in some forms of alopecia body hair is also affected). Women who have hirsutism(excess hair growth) on other parts of the body, together with acne and scalp hair loss are likely to have a hormonal imbalance. The overall state of the skin is important too.

Inflammation is a sign of infectious alopecia, while scarring and/or scaling may indicate lupus erythematosus or some other disorder. In alopecia areata, the nails are often pitted and ridged. The condition of the remaining hair is also revealing.

Broken off hairs may indicate trichotillomania, for example – a condition which is hard to detect by history-taking as patients tend to deny that they pull out their own hair. Sometimes the doctor will order some laboratory tests, especially if he suspects either a thyroid problem or anaemia.

Women with shedding hair should have both their serum iron checked (this is the usual test for anaemia), as well as their serum ferritin, which measures iron stores. A hormone profile is necessary for women who have scalp hair loss, hirsutism, and acne as they may have raised levels of the male hormone, testosterone. Blood tests may also be done to detect a scalp infection

What about the hair itself? A dermatologist or trichologist

may well carry out some further investigations. For instance, the likelihood of further hair loss can be assessed by grasping hold of a sample of eight to ten hairs and pulling on them. Only two hairs should come out if your hair is healthy; if four or more are are lost this indicates an abnormal level of shedding and the probability of further hair loss. Individual hairs can also be examined under the microscope.

This enables measurement of length, diameter, and growth phase. The bulb of a growing (anagen) hair is shaped differently to that of a resting (telogen) hair. The "gold standard" by which the health of the hair can be assessed is known as the unit area trichogram, developed by Hugh Rushton in the 1980's. The patient washes and combs their hair prior to the test using a standardised routine. Then a plastic template is placed on the scalp and a small circle marked on the skin with a felt tip pen.

Every hair within the circle is then plucked with forceps and mounted on a microscope slide. Various measurements can be made on this sample; the number of hairs, their length, and diameter, for example. The proportion in anagen and telogen can also be measured. One of the most useful measures to come out of the unit area trichogram is that of meaningful hair density.

Having a lot of hairs per unit area is not useful if they are very thin. The meaningful hair density is the number of hairs of greater than 40 micrometres diameter per unit area; this has been found to correlate well with cosmetically useful scalp coverage.

The unit area trichogram is extremely useful for assessing the progress of treatment, and in research for evaluating the efficacy of hair loss remedies (although, as we shall see in chapters 8 and 9, most remedies have not been subjected to this kind of investigation). However, as it is labour intensive, and invasive for the patient, the unit area trichogram is not used on a routine basis. Instead, many hair specialists use a phototrichogram; they will take a photograph of an area of scalp and make measurements from this.

An overview of hair loss treatments

The search for a cure for baldness goes back at least 5000 years, to remedies described in the papyri of ancient Egypt. The great Greek physician Hippocrates, working around 400BC, would prescribe opium mixed with essence of roses or lilies made into an ointment with wine, olive oil and acacia juice. For severe cases he recommended a paste of cumin, pigeon droppings, crushed horseradish and beetroot or nettles.

Some of the hair loss remedies on offer today are equally strange – such as curry paste, or Baby Bio rubbed into the scalp. The bottom line is that of all the products on the market, there is no sure-fire way of either growing back your hair, or of stopping further hair loss. Some types of hair loss require no treatment and will correct themselves with time, such as alopecia from cancer chemotherapy and, sometimes, alopecia areata. The treatments available for other kinds of hair loss fall into three main categories: tablets and lotions, wigs, and surgery.

Tablets and lotions

Genetic hair loss is thought to be caused by an inherited sensitivity of the hair follicles to the male sex hormone dihydrotestosterone (DHT). Anti-androgen drugs, which aim to block the action of DHT are effective in some cases of baldness.

They can be taken orally in women, but are generally rubbed into the scalp in men. The drawback is that they must be taken under medical supervision and may have side effects.

The only over the counter drug licensed for the treatment of genetic hair loss in men and women is minoxidil, sold as a 2 per cent solution known as Regaine®. Minoxidil causes hypertrichosis (excess hair growth) on the scalp but does not reverse hair loss. Many people see little or no benefit from minoxidil. In those who do, hair growth peaks within the first year, and treatment must be kept up indefinitely.

There are many other remedies on offer; few have been evaluated in a scientifically rigorous manner. In particular, lotions applied to the scalp do not have any effect on hair growth unless they reach the root. However, they may improve the appearance of the remaining hair.

There will undoubtedly be a chemical cure for genetic hair loss within the next few years. Drug companies have realised that baldness is an important quality of life issue for millions of men and women and therefore represents a huge market. Many are working on new anti-androgen type therapies. °For other forms of hair loss, the prescription depends upon the underlying condition. There are a number of drugs, such as steroids, which are commonly used in alopecia areata with varying degrees of success. (See chapter 8.)

Wigs

A cover-up in the form of a wig or hairpiece is a perfectly acceptable solution to any form of hair loss, particularly if it is temporary, such as anagen effluvium caused by chemotherapy.

Acrylic wigs are cheap and easy to look after. However, they do not always look very realistic, or fit well. A real hair wig is a better option, but is expensive and requires some care if you want it to carry on looking good. (See chapter 6)

Surgery

The scalp can be "rearranged" by surgery to minimise the balding area and maximise the hair bearing skin. The usual operation involves transfer of hair from the sides and back of the head to the hairline. Other types of surgery, such as removal of part of the bald area, are far less usual in the UK. Surgery is effective for genetic hair loss. In other cases, suitability varies and requires full assessment by a qualified person.

Drawbacks to surgery include its expense and the difficulty of finding a reputable surgeon – plus the risks of infection and so on which are inherent in any form of cosmetic surgery.

However the techniques of hair surgery are considerably more advanced than they were a decade ago and cosmetically acceptable results are possible. (See chapter 7)

And the rest

Some new directions in hair loss treatments include electric field therapy, various types of complementary medicine, and techniques for improving the blood supply to the scalp. None of these have been evaluated by the standard methods now available (such as the unit area trichogram discussed above). Which is not to say that they do not have some beneficial effect, but you would be wise not to expect too much – especially if you suffer from genetic hair loss. These alternative therapies are probably best for hair loss where stress is a precipitating factor. Some of these treatments are discussed in chapter 9.

Scalp cooling treatment in cancer chemotherapy

Doctors have known for over 20 years that cooling the scalp during chemotherapy can prevent alopecia. Cooling constricts the blood vessels in the scalp, which means that a lower dose of chemotherapy reaches the rapidly dividing cells in the hair follicles.

It also reduces activity of the hair cells, making them less vulnerable to the toxic effects of the drug. Reduction in alopecia is only seen if the scalp temperature falls below 22°C (from a normal body temperature of 37°C).

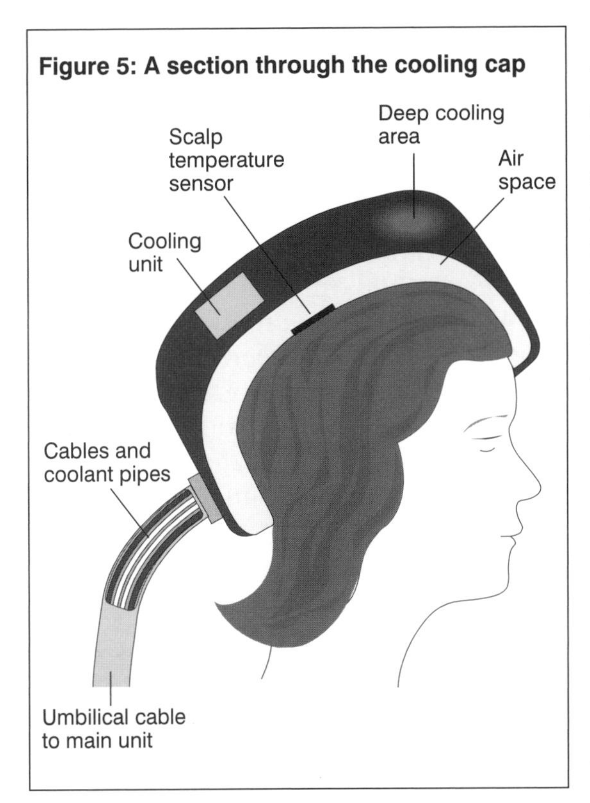

Figure 5: A section through the cooling cap

There are many ways of cooling the scalp to this temperature. The simplest is just to apply a cold cap, filled with ice, dry ice or a cooling gel. However, these can be heavy and uncomfortably cold for the patients. Nurses find them inconvenient because they have to be changed during the treatment (ice melts, and other coolants start to warm up). Over the last few years a number of cooling machines have been developed, such as the Scalp Cooling System II (SCS II). These circulate either cold air or a coolant liquid through a lightweight cap and are thermostatted so that the scalp stays at a constant temperature.

Clinical trials suggest that scalp cooling gives reasonable hair preservation in 50-70 per cent of patients. The outcome depends not upon which cooling system is used, but on the drugs used in the chemotherapy. Hair preservation is especially poor when a cocktail of drugs, such as cyclophosphamide, doxorubicin, and 5-fluorouracil, is used. However, when 39 women treated with docetaxel, a new drug for advanced breast cancer, used a cold cap results were very promising. Without scalp cooling 95 per cent of patients on docetaxol suffer grade 111 alopecia. With the cold cap, only one woman out of the total of 39 had hair loss to this extent. Twenty one of the women had no hair loss at all.

The availability of scalp cooling varies throughout the UK. Some hospitals have had the equipment for years (although they may not offer it routinely), while others have never heard of it. Caroline Woolfson, who suffered severe hair loss during intensive chemotherapy for ovarian cancer, has recently launched a charity called Headlines which is dedicated to raising money for machines like the SCS 11. A cooling machine has recently been delivered to the prestigious Christie Hospital in Manchester where it is being put through some clinical trials.

So if you are upset by the idea of losing your hair because of chemotherapy, do ask your specialist about scalp cooling.

Thanks to Headlines, the treatment is likely to become more widely available over the next few years. However, it is not suitable for every cancer patient. If you have leukaemia, for instance, it is important to keep up the level of chemotherapy everywhere in the blood circulatory system – including the scalp – because this is where the malignant cells are.[1]

Paying for hair loss treatments

Because most cases of hair loss are viewed by the medical profession as being a cosmetic rather than a clinical problem there is little treatment available on the National Health Service (NHS). People with cancer or alopecia areata can obtain subsidised or free wigs (see chapter 6 for details). Scalp cooling treatments during cancer chemotherapy are also paid for by the NHS where they are available.

The NHS does not, as a rule, pay for treatment by a

trichologist or hairdresser, or for hair loss surgery – for whatever reason. The same applies for most of the drug treatments and other remedies discussed in chapters 8 and 9, although a dermatologist may prescribe drugs such as steroids under the NHS for conditions like alopecia areata.

How to complain

Doctors and researchers are finally waking up to the fact that hair loss can seriously affect quality of life. The bogus clinics and cowboy operators have, unfortunately, been wise to this fact for many years. There are many products around which claim, on the basis of so-called "clinical research", a near 100 per cent track record in hair restoration. Anyone can call him or herself a hair specialist, qualified or not. And the only real barrier to setting yourself up as a hair surgeon is that it is illegal to have possession of the local anaesthetics and other drugs used in the operation unless you are medically qualified.

You are not required to have any kind of training before you relocate a large portion of someone's scalp from the back to the front of their head. Some dentists are, apparently, setting themselves up as hair transplant surgeons. They may be perfectly competent – but if the situation were reversed, you would probably think twice before letting a cosmetic surgeon fill or extract your teeth.

Yet few people actually complain about the false claims and shoddy treatment that abound in the world of hair loss treatment. The reasons are easy enough to understand. Consumers are reluctant enough to complain in general either because they blame themselves if things go wrong, or because they do not know how to go about lodging an effective protest. When it comes to a sensitive subject such as hair loss people are even less likely to complain because they just feel too embarrassed to admit that they sought treatment. The Trading Standards Authority, the Advertising Standards Authority, and the courts all admit they deal with very few cases concerning hair loss treatment. Which is a pity. Unless they are challenged, the bogus organisations will just continue to prey on vulnerable people.

If you are not satisfied with a hair loss treatment, take action. There are three aspects you can complain about: misleading advertising, products that do not perform to expectation, and actual harm caused by treatments such as surgery.[2, 3]

Advertising

The Advertising Standards Authority (ASA) encourages the public to report any advertisements in magazines, newspapers and leaflets delivered through the mail or from door-to-door which are not "legal, decent, honest and truthful". They also do their own spot checks. The ASA asks the company to produce evidence for the claims made in the ad. If it cannot do so, it will be asked to withdraw the advert and the case will be made public in the ASA's report. Most newspapers and magazines have agreed not to carry adverts if requested not to by the ASA. Here are some recent examples:

A tabloid newspaper carried an ad for a lotion said to contain hair growth formula which "is applied ... by massaging a few drops into the scalp daily until the desired effect is achieved". When challenged, the company could not produce any evidence for their claims about new hair growth. The ASA criticised both the company and the newspaper, and the ad was withdrawn.

A direct mail advert for hair restorer claimed it had been "successfully developed to regrow lost hair and stop further hair loss" and was "tried and tested by GMTV". It was accompanied by "before" and "after" pictures. The complainant wanted to know if these were genuine pictures. The company did not reply to the ASA's enquiries.

One so-called expert claimed to be a "renowned hair

specialist and lecturer with 25 years specialist study of male and female baldness at leading research laboratories and teaching hospitals in the UK, America and the far East." When his track record was challenged by a Fellow of the Institute of Trichologists, the "expert" had to admit to being a pharmacist who had published many articles but "these were not necessarily on hair loss" [4]

Useless products

If you buy yourself a hair loss remedy on the belief that it is going to be '86 per cent' effective, or whatever, and it does not do anything for you, complain. Make a note of all the facts, and write to the manufacturer and ask for your money back. Nine times out of ten this will resolve the problem (although the manufacturer may wriggle out of it by saying you were unfortunately one of the 4 per cent of non-responders). You can also report the matter to your local trading standards officer (contactable through your local authority, possibly under consumer protection or consumer services) as the company may have contravened the Trade Descriptions Act . They can prosecute and award you compensation (although cases involving hair loss treatments are extremely rare).[5]

Personal injury

If you have had hair surgery that has gone wrong, leaving you with say, an infection, or cosmetically unacceptable damage, you can try suing the surgeon or clinic. You will need to recruit an expert witness; the Institute of Trichologists can provide you with one.

You can get general consumer advice by joining the Consumer's Association who provide members with free legal advice. If you want to complain, but don't know where to begin , contact your local Citizen's Advice Bureau.

Further information

Books

Hair Loss: Coping with Alopecia Areata and Thinning Hair, Elizabeth Steel, Thorson's revised edition 1995 £6.99

How to Complain, Bridget Avison
Longman's Self-Help Guides, 1986

You and Yours How to Complain, David Berry
BBC Books, 1990

Trichology Clinics

The Scalp and Hair Clinic 108 St John's Hill
London SW11 1SY Tel:0171-924-2195

Philip Kingsley Trichological Clinic, 54 Green St
London W1Y 3RH Tel:0171-629-4004

Dr Hugh Rushton 22, Harley St, London W1
Tel:0171-637-4853

Organisations

The Institute of Trichologists 20-22 Queensberry Place
London SW7 2DZ Tel: 01625-862679

Send a large sae for a practitioner list and/or advice on litigation (mark your envelope either practitioner list or legal list)

Hairline International The Alopecia Patients' Society
Lyons Court 1668 High Street Knowle
West Midlands B93 0LY

Advice and support group for people with hair problems. Send a large sae for more information

The Advertising Standards Authority 2 Torrington Place
London WC1E 7HW Tel:0171-580-5555
Internet: http://www.asa.org.uk

The Consumers Association 2 Marylebone Rd,
London NW1 4BX Tel;0171-486 5544

BACUP 3 Bath Place, Rivington Street, London EC2A 3JR Cancer Information Service 0171-613-2121, or freephone 0800 18 11 99. BACUP is the leading national charity providing information and counselling for people affected by cancer.

Free leaflets available on chemotherapy and hair loss

Christie Hospital Appeals Tel. 0161-446-3988

Advises about the scalp cooling treatment and the Headlines appeal

Internet

The Bald Man's Home Page http://www.rebl.com/bald.html
The latest news from the US on transplant techniques and hair loss remedies and a chance to share your experiences. There's even a joke section.

Chapter 6

The big cover-up

Wigs go back a long way. The pharoahs of ancient Egypt shaved their heads so they could wear wigs as a sign of status, while slaves were made to keep their own hair as a reminder of their lowly caste. The custom spread to other cultures, and wig wearing reached peak popularity in 17th and 18th century Europe.

By this time, wigs were being worn not only as a fashion statement, but also as a cover-up for baldness.

The high status ceremonial wig now appears only in the courtroom (and the legal profession is even talking of giving up its traditional headgear). Wigs (or hairpieces as some people prefer to call them) for hair loss are now made to look as realistic as possible. A wig covers the whole head, while a toupee just covers the bald area. People with thin hair (who may not actually be suffering from alopecia) will often use a hair extension, which is just a hairpiece which adds length, body and volume. They are especially popular with performing artists who need a touch of glamour for the stage, or a change of image for a theatrical role.

For hair loss, wearing a hairpiece still has a slightly jokey image – maybe because an ill-fitting wig looks odd, and there is the potential embarrassment of having it fall or blow off. And some people who do cover up baldness with a wig hate to admit it.

But a hairpiece can be an excellent choice for anyone suffering from hair loss. Typically a wig retailer will fit people with alopecia areata, genetic hair loss, and with hair loss from cancer chemotherapy

There are two types of wig – acrylic and real hair. Both can look good, so long as you are prepared to look after them properly. Acrylic wigs are, by far, the cheaper option, but a hand-made real hair wig will fit better and be as close to your own hair as it is possible to get.

Acrylic wigs

Buying an acrylic wig is a bit like buying a hat – you just try it on and go for one that suits you. Acrylic wigs are made by machine in a number of styles, colours and sizes. There is no shortage of retailers specialising in acrylic wigs, and you can also buy by mail order. A good shop will let you try out their hairpieces in a private fitting room. Prices start at around £60. At this price you may be able to indulge in a whole wardrobe of wigs in different styles and colours.

At first I always got the same kind of wig – near to my original colour. Then I met my husband and he couldn't understand why I didn't turn wearing a wig to my advantage. So I went to a very trendy company and they suggested I go blonde. I felt really self-conscious at first, but everyone said how good it looked. So now I have different wigs all the time. I change them every day, and most people know I wear them. Eilidh, 27, clerical officer

The wig is kept in place by double-sided tape (known as toupee tape). It is not meant to be worn 24 hours a day; even the lightest wig feels hot and uncomfortable when worn in bed. If you do want to keep your naked scalp covered up, it's best to swop the wig for a cotton or light wool scarf, or perhaps a towelling turban, at night.

An acrylic wig is very easy to look after. It just needs to be washed in cold water with ordinary shampoo. A touch of fabric conditioner in the final rinse helps keep it looking good. It should then be left to dry naturally. Acrylic wigs should be kept away from all sources of heat such as hairdryers, heated rollers or curling tongs. It is not meant to be styled (choose the style when you buy it). The only hairdressing it needs is combing and perhaps a bit of hair spray. Cared for properly, a good quality wig should last around nine months.

Real hair wigs

Real hair wigs are made to measure by specialist companies. At your first consultation, the designer will discuss your requirements and give you some idea of how the wig will make you look.

If you decide to go ahead, the designer will next make a cast of your head using plastic sheeting and sellotape. At the same session he will also take measurements of your head. If you still have some hair, he will take a sample to match it for colour, texture and type (straight or curly). Otherwise, you should take along some photographs of yourself before you lost your hair.

While you can go for a completely new look, it may be wiser to ask your designer to create something that is as close to your original hair as possible. Losing your hair is shock enough, says designer Richard Mawbey, without finding that your expensive real hair wig just isn't 'you' when you look in the mirror. If you have set your heart on a different colour and texture from your original hair, it might be sensible to try it out with an acrylic wig first to see if you really can live with it.

The next stage is to order the hair for your wig from a hair merchant. Much of this comes from Eastern Europe, where many people are keen to sell their hair. Only human hair is used, as a rule, although yak hair is occasionally blended with human in a theatrical wig.

The foundation for the wig is also created, from the cast of the head. The most advanced foundations are made of a light terylene, which is very comfortable. You will then come in for a fitting of the foundation, and any final adjustments are made.

At this stage you will also be shown the hair which will be used to make the wig.

Then the wig is made by hand – which may take from three to six weeks. The wig maker will knot the hair into the foundation. When it is ready, the designer will fit the wig for you and together you will decide on the style. Usually the hair is left slightly on the long side, in case you want to alter the style and length later.

A real hair wig is fixed to the head with double-sided toupee tape (like an acrylic wig). If you have some hair, the wig can be attached to it with clips. The most advanced real hair wigs can be washed with shampoo and conditioner. Older style wigs use ribbons and springs in the foundation which should not get wet; these have to be dry cleaned, and this may alter the colour slightly.

When washing a real hair wig, it is important to keep it on a wig block, otherwise the foundation may shrink and the wig will not fit as well. There is also a danger of the knots of hair becoming loose. It will need to be washed every four to six weeks. The wig maker will do it for you, but it's quite possible to wash it for yourself if you live some distance away.

It can be styled, on the block, as if you were at the hairdressers, and final adjustments made on the head. But a real hair wig should not be coloured or permed as this may damage it.

A real hair wig will probably need to be replaced every two to three years. Many people keep a spare for when the other is being washed. An old wig can be refurbished by the addition of fresh hair. As you get older, it's sensible for the wig to grow old with you; that means going grey at a realistic rate.

Grey hair (which, incidentally, is the most expensive of all to buy) can be added gradually to an existing wig. This looks more natural than going grey overnight with a new wig.

A real hair wig costs £800 upwards. Adding hair to an existing wig will cost £50 to £100.[1]

I am about to get my fourth real hair wig. I had been wearing acrylic wigs for about 20 years. Then I moved to England and just happened to meet a wig maker who said 'Why do you wear such awful wigs?' He introduced me to Richard, who designs my wigs. Till then I had no idea there was any such thing as a real hair wig. There is no information for women about this sort of thing.

For me, the most amazing thing about them is that they just don't look like wigs. You don't have to worry about them blowing off. And you can even feel the wind blowing through your hair, which you can't with acrylic. My wig is very light, and it fits like a glove. I truly think people cannot tell I am wearing a wig.

My three wigs are all the same colour as my original hair, but at the same time they are different from each other. Number One is a bit frizzy, Number Two goes flat and Number Three is a bit shorter than the other two. I wear Number Three around the house, and Number One for business. Unfortunately Number Two is missing at the moment. At one time I thought Number One was dead because she began to look tired. But Richard has rejuvenated her by recolouring and adding more hair.

A real hair wig is more trouble than an acrylic wig. I wear a little cap at night. You really mustn't sleep in a wig as it gets pushed backwards. If you make love in the wig, it ends up looking like boiled wool. It gets all matted like a dog's coat.

The same thing happens if you even lean back on the headrest on a plane. It can recover but it's best not to treat it like that too often.

One really good thing about a real hair wig is that it makes you look younger. Womens' normal hair ages, but wig hair looks better than your own hair in every way. For presentation I think it makes you look better than you ever did. If you could only sleep in a real hair wig, I think it would be a total solution. Ann, 46 Business consultant.

Paying for wigs

Under certain circumstances the NHS will pay for, or pay towards, a wig. This usually happens if you have lost your hair from cancer chemotherapy, alopecia areata, or are having your head shaved for brain surgery. The consultant in charge of your case can prescribe a wig for you if he thinks it is necessary. People in hospital, children in school, and young people up to age 19 in full time education will get free wigs. So do people on income support or receiving family credit. People on low incomes may be entitled to financial help towards their prescription.

Otherwise, the NHS pays £45 towards an acrylic wig and £175 towards a real hair wig. You can be prescribed two acrylic wigs a year or two real hair wigs every three years (one to wear and one in the wash). In practice, hospitals tend to be rather reluctant to pay out for real hair wigs. Cancer patients may be able to get a grant towards a wig from the Cancer Relief Macmillan Fund, although application has to be made through a doctor or social worker. Value added tax (VAT) does not have to be paid by cancer patients but you have to complete the VAT form at the time of buying the wig as it cannot be claimed back later.[2, 3]

Hair weaving, bonding and 'liquid skin'

These are all methods of combining your existing hair with 'new' hair. Hair weaving was first developed in the 1960s. It involves plaiting existing hair in tight rows across the scalp and using these as a base to attach acrylic or real hair. Alternatively a fine net with hair attached can be placed on the scalp and the existing hair woven into this. The weaving has to be really tight, which may lead to traction alopecia.

In hair bonding, a plastic skull cap with 'new' hair is placed on the head and the existing hair pulled through tiny holes in its surface. The 'old' and 'new' hair can be glued or bonded together. Unlike a wig, you cannot easily remove a hair weave or bond and it may be far from comfortable.

Liquid hair is a thin transparent mesh onto which replacement hair is attached one strand at a time. The mesh can be attached to the scalp by a layer of silicone which is supposed to make it feel like a second skin. These developments are fairly recent, and it may be wise to consult a qualified trichologist before you decide to try them.

Further information

BACUP 'Coping with Hair Loss' has basic advice about wigs and NHS guidelines. Booklet available from the contact address given in chapter 5

Wig Specialties 173 Seymour Place, London W1H 5TP
Tel:0171-262-6565

Makes high quality real hair wigs.

Chapter 7

Surgery

Surgery offers the possibility of a permanent solution to your hair loss problem. It does not come cheap, and it can be hard to find a skilled and reputable surgeon. But techniques have improved dramatically over the last few years and there is no reason why you shouldn't expect to get a reasonable result. Hair surgery involves rearranging your scalp skin so as to minimise the bald bits and maximise the remaining hair-bearing areas. There are two basic techniques – grafts and flaps. In the UK, most hair surgeons use grafts; in the United States both techniques are on offer. Surgery is applicable to genetic hair loss in both men and women. It may also be successful in other forms of hair loss. Grafting became established in the Western world in the late 1950s (although the first report came from Japan in 1939), while flap surgery is more recent, dating from 1977.

Hair grafting

A graft is a piece of skin which is transferred from one part of the body to another, without its original blood supply. Any piece of tissue without a blood supply will eventually die. So the success of a skin graft relies on the development of a new blood supply in the recipient site. Until this happens, the graft obtains nutrients and oxygen by diffusion from surrounding tissue. A hair graft is a specialised type of skin graft; it involves the transfer of skin from the hair-bearing areas of the scalp (known as the donor site) to the bald area (which is known as the recipient site).

People often call this kind of operation a hair transplant.

Perhaps this is a little bit misleading. Most other transplant surgery involves transferring an organ such as a heart, liver or kidney, from a donor to a recipient. Normally the immune system would reject a such a 'foreign' organ. Patients undergoing organ transplant surgery only get away with it by taking powerful drugs to suppress the immune system for the rest of their lives.

If you received someone else's hair, your scalp would reject it. You may have heard of implant surgery. This involves inserting synthetic hair into a balding area of scalp. No reliable trichologist recommends hair implant surgery as it usually leads to infection.

A hair graft is a transplant only in the gardening sense. It is a bit like transplanting seedlings or a shrub. Your own hair is the plant, and the scalp is the garden. You have to use your own hair for the graft. The crucial question is whether you still have enough hair to make the operation successful.

Hair grafts work because of a phenomenon called donor dominance. The transplanted hair retains its own characteristics (that is, it grows) rather than that of the scalp it is transferred to (which cannot grow useful hair). So the hair graft keeps on growing, despite being on what appears to be an unproductive area of the scalp. It is well established that donor dominance occurs in genetic hair loss. If you are considering surgery for another type of hair loss, it is up to your surgeon to assess whether it is of the donor dominant type or not. For instance, in the scarring alopecia that occurs with lupus erthematosus (see chapter 2) a graft takes on the characteristics of the underlying bald scalp and will not grow hair (this is known as recipient dominance)

If hair grafts are greater than four millimetres in diameter, diffusion of nutrients and oxygen from surrounding tissue – which the graft depends on prior to establishing its own blood supply – is very inefficient. So the grafts usually die long before they can produce any new hair from lack of nourishment. Grafts of around three millimetres diameter – just at the upper limit of viability – were the norm until a few years ago. These grafts usually carry between eight and 30 hairs and are known as punch, round or cylindrical grafts. A single or double row of punch grafts is removed from a hair bearing area – commonly the back of the head – by a cylindrical cutter (see figure 6 below). The surgeon then makes some holes of a slightly smaller diameter in the balding area of the scalp and 'plugs' in the grafts one by one. It is usual to set the grafts in a chequerboard style over four sessions to give each set a chance to establish its own blood supply. Making the recipient holes a little smaller in diameter than the donor holes ensures a good fit; the surrounding skin tends to shrink up around the graft.

Unfortunately surgery using only plug grafts gives an unnatural tufted appearance, rather like doll's hair. The effect can be particularly bad around the hairline where the

Figure 6. Donor grafts are often taken from the hair-bearing area at the back of the head

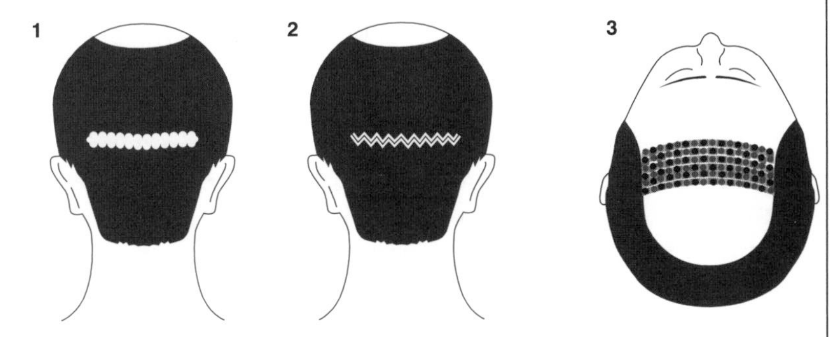

Either a single or double row of plug grafts, or a single strip, is cut out (1), and the area is then stitched up (2). The plug grafts are positioned in four separate grafting sessions across the area to be covered (3). Spacing the grafts allows their new blood supply to develop.

transition from the bare forehead to the transplanted hair is just too abrupt. But you don't have to put up with this any more, thanks to the advent of mini- and micrografts. These, as the name suggests, are much smaller pieces of hair-bearing skin than the plug graft. A minigraft will be one to three millimetres in diameter, containing just three to six hairs. And a micrograft is smaller still and may contain only one hair. Minigrafts may be punched direct from the hair bearing area. Alternatively, the surgeon may cut a strip of skin (typically ten cm long and up to one and a half centimetres wide) from, say, the back of your head and dissect out hundreds of minigrafts. A micrograft is always dissected out from a bigger piece of graft.

Minigrafts and micrografts are used to create a natural looking hair line, and to fill in spaces between plug grafts.

They are especially good for women with diffuse hair loss, where plug grafts would just look silly. Strategic placing of mini or micrografts in thinning hair will create an acceptably dense look.

The surgeon makes either tiny slits or pinholes in the recipient area for the placement of mini and micrografts. Although these small holes cause less trauma to the scalp they do not, like plug graft holes, remove bald skin. So they do not give such dense coverage as plug grafts. Increasingly, however, hair surgeons and their clients are realising that a natural look is more acceptable, in the long run, than dense coverage. Incidentally, you may have heard of lasers being used in transplant surgery. While this sounds advanced (like the use of lasers to remedy short sight), it turns out that lasers have not fulfilled their early promise as they tend to damage the grafts. Also lasers are very expensive. So if your surgeon proposes to use an ordinary scalpel for your surgery, do not be disappointed.

Two factors will affect the way your surgeon plans your graft.

The first is the amount of hair available for grafting, and the second is the extent of future hair loss – which will increase the bald area over time. Each case is unique, but if you do not have enough hair for transplanting to both your hairline and your crown – while keeping some in reserve to cover future losses – then most surgeons will advise building up your hairline. This is because a natural hairline creates a frame for your face, making you look younger. Loss of hair from the crown happens in nearly all men as they get older and is not nearly as obvious as a receding hairline.

To build up a hairline, you should have micrografts at the front, and either plug or minigrafts (or a mixture) a few rows back. This creates a natural looking graduation in density. For this the surgeon might insert a minimum of, say, up to 300 micrografts and maybe the same number of minigrafts. You may get a reasonable result with just one session of grafting – or you may need several more.[3, 4]

Case histories

People's experience of hair surgery varies enormously. Steve went to a commercial clinic over ten years ago, and has now consulted a registered trichologist for advice on repair work.

John is still having work done by a doctor who is a Fellow of the Royal College of Surgeons.

I saw a dermatologist at the hospital, and he said I'd just have to grin and bear it. Then this transplant clinic had an exhibition locally. The results looked good, although the guy who signed me up was a bit of a used salesman type. The clinic was a pretty plush place, I noticed.

First they injected my scalp at the front and back. That did hurt a bit. Then he cut out the hair at the back. I felt wetness and knew I was bleeding. Then they plugged it into the front. After, they bound my scalp up quite tight and suggested I took paracetamol for the pain. I did have a pretty bad headache for a couple of days, two black eyes, and my forehead was all swollen. I had four days off work but even then people noticed something was up. I hadn't told anyone about the transplant – only my parents.

Over the next two years, I had four consultations and they put more hair in at each session. But the disillusion set in after the first operation. I'd expected it to look more natural than it did. They kept saying they'd get it right, but in the end I decided enough damage had been done, so I stopped. Then the rest of my hair started to recede and a gap has opened up between that and my transplant. I tried 2 per cent minoxidil, that the same clinic sold me. Then I was prescribed 4 per cent minoxidil, and progesterone. They didn't do much good either. I tried a trichologist who gave me high frequency treatment, and massaged my scalp with a menthol solution. In all I've probably spent around £3000.

In a pub or a bar, people will stare, or make comments. Maybe a group of lads will say something, and I'll just have to leave. If there's something unusual about your appearance, people will always have a second look at you.

It wouldn't matter to me now if I was as bald as Duncan Goodhew – in fact, I'd be delighted. It's the transplant, rather than the hair loss, that upsets me now. And I can't get rid of it without doing more damage – apparently shaving would leave marks, and electrolysis would cause scarring. Still, I have decided to try and remedy the situation – perhaps with a repair of the transplant.

I suppose I was naive, but I do have a very bitter opinion of the company that did the transplant. I feel they misled me, and really fell down badly on the counselling side. But they still advertise in the papers, showing all these pictures of good looking men. Steve, 35, computer programmer

I was introduced to my hair surgeon by my brother, and that was lucky because there are more bad guys than good

guys out there. I've just come back from another session and I've had 350 grafts done. It was a piece of cake. It's all done and healing nicely. Basically I just feel a lot better about myself.

I start by being given a mild sedative, and I also get a prescription for antibiotics and drugs to stop swelling for the next few days. Then I go to the cutting room, which is basically like being at the hairdressers. The doctor cuts the hair from the donor area. Then I go into a dentist's type chair and get a shot of Valium. That makes you feel very relaxed – like being drunk but not completely out of it. Otherwise you would feel anxious, especially if it was your first time. Then I have injections of local anaesthetic which feel a bit sharp, but it's not a real problem. They take the donor area and divide it up, then decide what to use. Then they make incisions in the scalp and put the hair in.

The whole thing might take two to three hours. As far as bleeding goes there's not much. I might feel a little drop trickling down the side, that's all. Then I go to the recovery room and wait till the anaesthetic wears off and let the grafts settle. They say you should take it easy for the next day or so – no drinking, or sex, for instance. If you've still got hair, you will look fine. If you're bald, the scabs will be visible.

I went for surgery because I'm a musician and felt my hair loss was too visible on stage. Now I do feel more confident. I'm happy to talk to people who are thinking of seeing my doctor but are a bit anxious about the whole thing. I do feel for people who've got the problem of hair loss. I think it's always best to deal direct with the surgeon. You get agents touting for business, offering loans and it turns out the cost is twice what I pay. I've even been asked to say I had my hair done by some of these people. I could take the money and run, of course, but it's not right. My surgeon doesn't advertise – he doesn't need to. If he left the country I don't know what I'd do, because I wouldn't want anyone else to touch me. John, 46, musician

Hair flaps

Unlike grafts, skin flaps are transferred from one part of the body to another with their blood supply intact. As far as hair surgery is concerned, the flap operation most often carried out is a scalp reduction (see figure 7 below), clinically known as an advancement flap. A spindle-shaped flap is removed from the bald area (and then discarded, rather than being transferred elsewhere). As the scalp is somewhat elastic, the surrounding hair bearing areas can be 'pulled up' around the

Figure 7
Scalp reduction

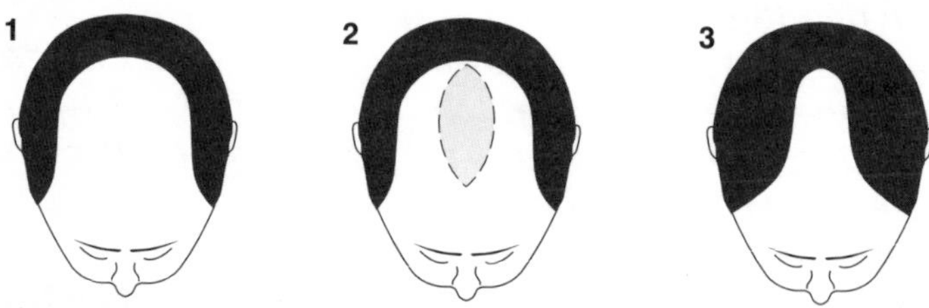

A piece of scalp is cut away from the top of the head (2), and the hair-bearing area stretched to its margins, minimising the bald area (3).

Scalp expansion

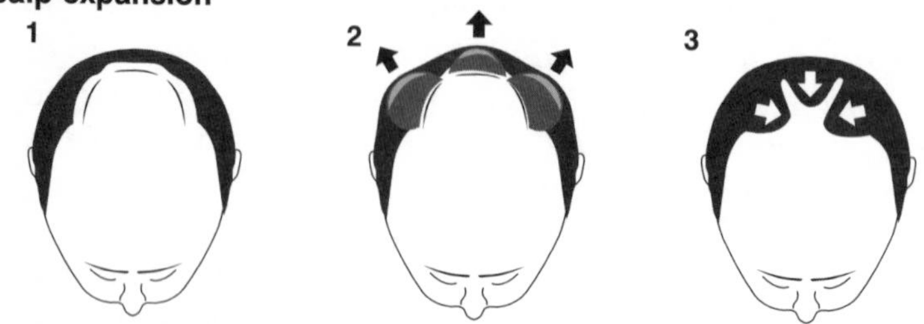

Incisions are made around the bald area (1), and silicone balloons inserted beneath the hair-bearing areas (2). These expand the overlaying skin and so extend the hairy scalp over the bald region, which is then removed (3).

flap area. One session may be all that is needed, especially if the scalp is elastic and the bald area small. Otherwise the process can be repeated after an interval of around four months. In people with a tight scalp, a flap of up to three centimetres in width can be removed at one time. But if your scalp is more elastic the surgeon might be able to remove a piece up to eight centimetres wide. Scalp reduction has always been more popular in the United States than it has here. And even in the States it has been in decline – at least until recently. There are, however, signs that scalp reduction may be coming back into favour again, at least on the West Coast.

There are a couple of related developments that have originated in the US. Scalp extensions stretch out the hair bearing areas of the scalp over the bald part. Silicone balloons are inserted under the scalp and then slowly inflated by the injection of sterile saline. The scalp lying over it then stretches and, at the same time, its cells divide more rapidly, creating new skin. Once the stretched scalp has expanded over the bald area, the latter is cut out. A really clever surgeon would then repair the join with a strip of hair-bearing scalp

All right, it sounds weird. In fact scalp expansion has perfectly feasible origins. Think how a skin of a pregnant woman expands to accommodate a growing foetus. And the process is well established for covering up head and neck burns. It is also used to help women who have lost a breast to cancer. If the skin of the chest wall is expanded over the site of the breast a 'pocket' for an artificial breast can be created.

The most recent development is the scalp extender. This is a device placed under the skin which expands the hair bearing area. But unlike the balloons mentioned above, it remains flat during the process – so the patient does not have to spend weeks hiding a bulging scalp. Combined with scalp reduction, this is said to be capable of removing large areas of bald scalp on the crown.[3, 4, 5]

Step-by-step through hair surgery

At the first, and possibly second, meeting with your surgeon you should discuss the following:

- ❑ your medical history
- ❑ what surgery can do for you, and your expectations
- ❑ the quality of your donor site, and your hair type
- ❑ your hair loss, and how it may progress over the years.

Medically speaking, most people can have hair loss surgery although people with heart disease, hypertension (high blood pressure) and diabetes may be viewed with some caution by the surgeon. Men with bleeding disorders such as haemophilia are not suitable candidates for surgery.

The surgeon should make clear to you that surgery will not give you back the head of hair you had before losing it. It is, in no sense, a baldness reversal process. The best that can be hoped for is to maintain an acceptable hair density as you get older.

It is also important to realise that this is not a one-off procedure. You may need further sessions over the years to keep up with increasing hair loss. Much depends on how the surgery is planned. The last thing you want is to end up with an unflattering gap between your transplant and the remaining hair as you go bald in later years. For some younger men who stand to lose a lot more hair, maybe the best decision is to defer surgery for a few years. By that time, they may have outgrown the wish for the operation when they see that most of their contemporaries are beginning to lose their hair. The result you can expect depends also on your hair type.

The ideal transplant patient would be a 50 year old Afro-Caribbean. At his age he will probably not lose too much more hair, and curly hair – when transplanted – gives better coverage than straight hair. The worst candidate is the 20 year old with straight, fair hair. But even he may get good results in the hands of a skilled surgeon.

Remember, this is a two way process, so be sure to quiz your surgeon. Take a friend or relative if that makes you feel more confident. Ask him how many operations he has done.

Surgeons learn their trade by watching their seniors carry out operations and then trying them out for themselves. You are about to make a substantial financial investment. He has to start somewhere but you'd probably prefer not to be his first patient.

A good surgeon will be only too happy to provide you with evidence of his skills; photographs, videos and – best of all – the phone numbers of past patients are immensely useful. Once you have decided to go ahead, you and your surgeon will discuss your proposed new hairline. It shouldn't be too far forward; not only will this look unnatural as you age, it will also use up too much of your remaining hair. On the other hand, starting it too far back from your forehead will give a flat unnatural look. He can use computers, diagrams or even a felt tip pen on your forehead to work out where the new hairline should be. Then he should talk you through your operation and give you leaflets to take away. You should feel free to phone with any questions you have before the day of the surgery.

Before the operation you should plan to have the hair at the back of your head long enough (a couple of centimetres, perhaps) to cover the donor area. You should also arrange to take a week off work and do not schedule any important engagements for this time. Most people recover in a day or so, but you cannot be sure how the surgery will affect you.

On the day of the operation you will normally be given a tranquilliser such as Valium about half an hour beforehand to quell any anxiety. You may also be given other drugs such as a vasoconstrictor to minimise bleeding, antibiotics, and perhaps steroids to control swelling after surgery. Then the surgeon will clip the hair in the donor area to within two millimetres of your scalp. You then receive injections of local anaesthetic into both the donor and recipient site.

A strip of hair (or a row of plug grafts) will then be removed from the back of your head. The area is then stitched.

Usually these stitches are the self-dissolving kind. The surgeon, working with an assistant, will dissect up a skin graft and then make the necessary holes in the area to be grafted.

Working with a microscope, they will then insert several hundred of the grafts over a period of up to four hours. After the operation you will wait in a recovery room for a while to check there is no unnecessary bleeding, before going home to rest. People vary in the amount of post-operative pain they experience. Usually it is controllable with a couple of paracetamol or a stronger over-the-counter painkiller like Nurofen Plus. Some surgeons may prescribe you a painkiller and sleeping pills for the first night or so. The donor area will be more sore than the recipient area.

Scabs form around the transplanted follicles. These usually fall off within a week or so, taking the transplanted hair with them. Do not panic. The transplanted follicle remains and should produce new hair around 12 weeks after the operation.

You will have to treat the transplanted area gently for a while. You can shampoo it gently in a few days (or as directed by the surgeon), but should not use combs and brushes on it for up to two weeks.

Serious side effects are rare. There is always a risk of infection with any form of surgery, but this can be minimised by following your surgeon's instructions carefully. One in 50 patients experiences some swelling or even black eyes for a few days after the operation. You may also notice a lack of sensation in the donor area. This should disappear after a while, but very occasionally it does become permanent.[1, 2]

How to find a hair surgeon

Finding a reputable and skilled surgeon is not easy. More and more people are setting up in business in the wake of the new mini and micrografting techniques. Some will have had very little experience. The best don't advertise much (they don't need to). The best way is probably by personal recommendation, through the Institute of Trichologists (see chapter 5 for the address) or through the recently launched British Association of Hair Restoration Surgeons (see below). Look for qualifications:

FRCS (Fellow of the Royal College of Surgeons), BAAPS (British Association of Aesthetic Plastic Surgeons), BACS(British Association of Cosmetic Surgeons), ISAPS (International Society of Aesthetic Plastic Surgeons), ISHRS (International Society of Hair Restoration Surgery). Having said that, the BAAPS appears to disapprove of hair restoration surgery, unless it is done for strictly clinical reasons, and will not give recommendations. The Royal College of Surgeons will not be able to advise you as they deal only with NHS work.

Further information

The British Association of Hair Restoration Surgeons
101 Princess St
Manchester M1 6DD

The intelligent man's guide to hair transplants and other methods of hair replacement, Walter P Unger & Sidney Katz, Contemporary Books, 1979. Out of print, but worth asking your library to obtain it. Dr Unger is one of the world's leading authorities.

Chapter 8

Chemical cures

There is, as yet, no pill or lotion which is guaranteed to give you back your hair. But there are some drugs that can give worthwhile results in various forms of hair loss. Most of them are only available on prescription. A trichology clinic may also offer topical solutions of anti-androgens (see below) without a prescription.

There are also numerous over-the-counter remedies for hair loss which you can get from a health food shop, a pharmacy, hair salons, or by mail order. Only one of these, Regaine®, is actually licensed for the treatment of hair loss. When a drug has a licence, it generally means that it has gone through extensive clinical trials which show the authorities (in the UK, the Medicines Control Agency, in the US, the Food and Drug Administration) that they are safe and effective.

This is not to say that the unlicensed remedies are necessarily useless. Clinical trials are expensive and time-consuming and small companies are not always able to undertake them. Some have done more limited research. But some companies would not want to put their hair loss remedies to the test for the simple reason that they would fail. So beware of extravagant claims such as '98 per cent success in 20 years of clinical research'. Ten to one the company would not be able to back these claims with hard evidence if challenged. We will take another look in chapter 9 at some of the unlicensed remedies that might be worth a try. Here we will look at anti-androgens, Regaine®, and some prescription drugs for alopecia areata.

Anti-androgen drugs

Genetic hair loss, though still not completely understood, is thought to result from an inherited over-sensitivity of the hair follicle to the androgen (male hormone) dihydrotestosterone (DHT). Therefore using drugs which block the action of DHT – anti-androgens – is a rational way of treating the condition. Anti-androgen therapy has indeed had some success in arresting or even reversing genetic hair loss in men and women.[12]

Some of the drugs in current use are listed in table 5 below.

TABLE 5

Anti-androgen drugs used to treat genetic hair loss*

- **Prednisone (Decortisyl)**
- **Dexamethasone (Decadron)**
- **Spironolactone (Aldactone)**
- **Ketoconazole (Nizoral)**
- **Cyproterone acetate**
- **Ethinyloestrodiol**
- **Flutamide (non-steroidal anti-androgen, still under investigation)**
- **Bromocriptine(Parlodel)**
- **Progesterone**

* in general, the anti-androgens are used topically in men and orally in women

Men given oral **medroxyprogesterone acetate** (a synthetic progesterone, and the active ingredient in DepoProvera, the injectable female contraceptive) effectively reversed their baldness in one unpublished study. But progesterone is a female sex hormone and while some synthetic versions are anti-androgenic, they may also have feminising side effects. For most men, the prospect of taking drugs akin to oral contraceptives or HRT is only marginally more appealing than castration – the only sure fire cure for male pattern baldness (see chapter 1).

Cyproterone acetate (CPA), also a synthetic progesterone, is a very potent anti-androgen and has been used with some success as a scalp lotion on men, as have some of the other drugs in table 5. CPA can certainly stop further hair loss, but will not regrow hair. Anti-androgen therapy – topical or oral – should only be given under medical supervision, preferably by an endocrinologist (hormone specialist) or a dermatologist with an interest in hormones. In other words, you should be monitored for side effects. Even if you are only rubbing the solution into the scalp, some absorption into the rest of the body may occur.

Cyproterone acetate (CPA) and ethinyl oestrodiol (EE) are the active ingredients of the oral contraceptive Dianette which is prescribed to women with acne and hirsutism resulting from an excess of male hormone. However, the amount of CPA in Dianette appears to be insufficient to treat female genetic hair loss.

Hugh Rushton and Ian Ramsay showed, in 1992, that giving women 50 mg of CPA from day one to day 15 of the menstrual cycle, along with EE from day 5 to day 24, was more effective than using Dianette. However, women whose iron stores were depleted (see chapter 2) did not experience significant hair growth. Those whose serum ferritin (a measure of total body iron stores) were greater than 40 micrograms/litre had an average increase of 20 per cent in useful hair density, while those with serum ferritin below this had only a 1 per cent increase. The untreated controls also showed differences in the amount of hair they lost – those with low serum ferritin lost more hair than those with adequate iron stores (table 6 opposite).[10, 11]

TABLE 6

Importance of serum ferritin in treatment of female androgenetic alopecia with oral cyproterone acetate and ethinyl oestrodiol (data from D.H.Rushton and I.D Ramsay, Clinical Endrocrinology, 1992, 36,421-427)

Change in useful hair density	
Treated	
◆ Women with adequate serum ferritin	+20 per cent
◆ Women without adequate serum ferritin	+1 per cent
Untreated	
◆ Women with adequate serum ferritin	-7 per cent
◆ Women without adequate serum ferritin	-10 per cent

Minoxidil (Regaine®)

Regaine® consists of a 2 per cent solution of the drug minoxidil in a solution of ethanol, propylene glycol and water and is designed to be applied to the scalp.

Minoxidil was originally developed, in tablet form, as a medication for high blood pressure by the pharmaceutical company Upjohn Limited, of Kalamazoo, Michigan (the company has since merged and is now known as Pharmacia & Upjohn Inc). Minoxidil lowers blood pressure by acting as a vasodilator – a drug which opens up the blood vessels, making it easier for the blood to flow through. In the late 1960s, doctors began to notice that minoxidil had a curious side effect – patients taking it began to grow new hair. A clinical report in the New England Journal of Medicine described a 38-year-old man with kidney disease who had lost much of his hair when he was 20. Within four weeks of starting minoxidil, dark brown hair (his original colour) began to grow on his bald scalp. This new hair was similar in thickness and texture to his original hair. By the time he left hospital, after 16 weeks of treatment, the new hair was an inch long – enough to make it look as if his baldness had been reversed.[7]

Upjohn went on to develop minoxidil as a treatment for hair loss. In 1983, the company launched the first ever large-scale study of male pattern baldness, involving around 3000 men, aged between 18 and 49, suffering from moderate hair loss (Hamilton Scale III, IV and V – see figure 3, page 13). The men took part in a double-blinded placebo-controlled clinical trial of 2 per cent and 3 per cent minoxidil solution. They were divided into three groups: two received either 2 per cent or 3 per cent minoxidil, while the third, control, group received the placebo, which was just the liquid that is used to make up the minoxidil solution. The double-blinding means that neither the investigators or the men involved know which lotion they were using. This technique is standard in clinical trials, and is meant to eliminate bias so the product is tested fairly.

The men rubbed 1 ml of lotion into the balding area twice a day, and most kept up the treatment for a full year. By this time, 68 per cent of the men had minimal to moderate regrowth, while in 8 per cent the regrowth was said to be thick. For the rest, minoxidil did at least stop any further hair loss, even if no new hair grew. There was no significant difference between 2 per cent and 3 per cent minoxidil, while concentrations less than 2 per cent were ineffective.[15]

However, the methods used for assessing the hair regrowth have been severely criticised so it is probably as well not to put too much faith in the above figures.

Regaine® has also been tested on women with genetic hair loss, in a trial which is generally better regarded by those in the know than the male trial described above. Two hundred and fifty six women with hair loss corresponding to Ludwig took part in a trial of 2per cent minoxidil. The investigators reported that 63 per cent of the women had minimal to moderate regrowth of their hair at the end of the trial period and the results are described in table 7 below. [13]

TABLE 7

Clinical trial of minoxidil in women with alopecia androgentica

Time in weeks	2% minoxidil 128 patients	placebo 128 patients
0	Av. hair count*140	139
8	157	145
32	163	148
Dermatologist estimated hair growth **		
dense	0	0
moderate	13	6
minimal	50	33
Patient estimated hair growth		
dense	0	0
moderate	20	7
minimal	40	33

* The average hair count was for a one cm square of scalp

** Both dermatologist and patient evaluated hair regrowth in this study; data are percentages of patients in each group

Regaine® is only licensed for the treatment of genetic hair loss in men and women. A doctor may prescribe it for other forms of hair loss, if he thinks it appropriate, but he – rather than the company – then bears the responsibility for its use. It has been tested for alopecia areata; a 3 per cent solution of minoxidil gave some hair growth in 36 per cent of patients in one trial, while a 5 per cent solution produced regrowth in 54 per cent of the group. In another trial, 5 per cent minoxidil – used over a 60-week period – regrew hair in 86 per cent of patients with severe alopecia areata. It sounds impressive but what the researchers downplay in this report is that the regrowth was only 'cosmetically acceptable' in 6 per cent of their patients. In other words, the rest still needed to use wigs or hats to disguise their baldness. In alopecia areata, minoxidil may be more useful if used in conjunction with steroid treatment, as discussed below.[9]

Regaine® is available from chemists. As it is classed as a 'pharmacy' medicine, it can only be sold on premises where a pharmacist is present. You cannot buy Regaine® from health food shops, or supermarkets. And in the chemist's it is kept behind the counter, rather than on open shelves.

Before selling Regaine® a pharmacist should ask: who is it for? Is that person taking any medication? If so, what for? Is there any history of high blood pressure or thyroid problems? What age is the patient? People with high blood pressure should only use Regaine® under a doctor's supervision. Regaine® costs £24.95 for a month's supply (one 60 ml bottle). Five per cent solutions of Regaine® are available on private prescription at £30 for 30 days' supply. Do not pay large sums to private hair clinics for Regaine®.

What kind of results can you expect from Regaine®? Expect to wait for up to four months before anything happens. If you have had no response after six months to a year it is not worth continuing with the treatment. Based on all the clinical trials so far, the manufacturers say one third of men will get good hair growth, while another third get a fine, downy regrowth. The remaining third will get little or no response.

Younger men, those who have been balding for a only short time or who only have a small bald patch tend to do best; however, it is impossible to predict individual responses. You may find that the hair that grows initially is vellus hair and that later it seems to become thicker and more like your normal hair. At least part of this might be due to the fact that Regaine® appears to coat the hair shafts, making them look thicker and darker. The majority of men will find that at least they do not lose any more hair. Regaine® is at least as successful –

sometimes more so – in women.

Once you decide to give Regaine® a go, it is important to stick to the twice daily routine. And you will have to use it indefinitely. Once you stop, the new hair falls out after 3 to 4 months and the balding process will continue.[1, 4, 6]

Steroids

The steroids are a category of biologically active compounds which include the sex hormones, and other hormones involved in the mineral, fluid and sugar balance of the body. The anabolic steroids, which are used (often illegally) in sport, build muscle and increase strength and stamina. Medically, however, their main use is to damp down inflammation. The immune system produces an inflammatory response – pain, swelling and heat – whenever the body is under threat, say, from infection. This is all well and good. But from time to time, the immune system starts up inflammation when it is not helpful, resulting in diseases such as arthritis, asthma and allergy. Because alopecia areata is thought to result from the immune system attacking the hair follicles (see chapter 2), treatment with steroids such as prednisone may be helpful. For less severe cases of alopecia areata (less than 60 per cent hair loss) steroids such as betamethasone (Betnovate) cream may be prescribed to rub into the scalp nightly. Small patches of baldness may also respond to injections of cortisone into the affected area.

Where hair loss is really extensive, a dermatologist might consider putting a patient on oral steroids – typically, prednisone (Decortsyl) – for a short time, but usually only if topical treatments with steroids and other drugs have been unsuccessful. This is not a decision to be taken lightly, as potential side effects include mood swings, weight gain and, in the longer term, a greater susceptibility to hypertension, diabetes and osteoporosis. Unfortunately, the regrown hair tends to fall out once the steroids are stopped. But if they are continued long-term, the risk of troublesome side effects increases. To get patients out of this double-bind situation, some dermatologists are now offering combination therapy. In a typical combination treatment programme, a short course of steroids is used to regrow a decent amount of hair. It is then followed up by long-term minoxidil to make sure the hair growth is sustained.

In a trial carried out in 1992 at Duke University Medical Centre, North Carolina, by Elise Olsen and her team, 32 patients with alopecia areata took small doses of prednisone for six weeks. Half of the group had either alopecia totalis or alopecia universalis. At the end of the steroid treatment,15 patients had significant regrowth (in eight regrowth was complete).

These results are much better, for the same time period, than any other treatment for alopecia areata. There were some minor side effects from the steroids (mainly weight gain or mood swings) but these were not bad enough to cause any patient to drop out of the trial.

Then the patients were divided into two groups and randomly assigned to either 2 per cent minoxidil or placebo for five months. At the end of this time nearly half the patients in the minoxidil group had retained, or even increased, their hair growth, compared to none in the placebo group.[14, 2]

Other drugs for alopecia areata

Topical immunotherapy involves rubbing an irritating substance into the scalp in the hope that it will direct the attention of the immune system away from the hair follicles. If it works, the patient will get dermatitis on the affected area – a sign that the immune system is responding to the irritant. The drugs used are known as contact sensitisers. The three which have been tried are dinitrochlorobenzene (DNCB), squaric acid dibutyl ester (SADBE), and diphenylcyclopropenone (diphencyprone, DPCP).

Results are variable, but are generally reckoned to be as good as steroids and without the side effects. Thirty to 40 per cent of patients had regrowth in some trials. DPCP seems to be superior to SADBE. There is some concern over the safety of DNCB. Laboratory tests have suggested it could cause cancer, but this is controversial.

Anthralin (Dithranol), a tar-based cream used in psoriasis, has had some success in the treatment of alopecia areata, particularly in combination with minoxidil. It is known as a contact irritant and appears to work in a broadly similar way to topical immunotherapy.

Another treatment often used for psoriasis which has some application to alopecia areata is PUVA (psoralen plus ultraviolet A) therapy. It is a form of light therapy; patients take a drug called psoralen (derived from plant extracts) which sensitises their bald area to the application of long-wavelength ultra-violet light. The treatment is time-consuming – requiring up to five sessions a week, and a total of 20 before any regrowth can be expected.

Recent evidence suggests that hair usually falls out again if PUVA is discontinued. Of 70 patients, 50 per cent regrew some hair during the treatment period, but only 15 per cent kept the hair if they then stopped. The problem with long term PUVA is that ultra-violet light is ageing, and may also cause cancer. There has also been some limited use of immune suppressant drugs for alopecia areata, working on the idea that if the immune system could be damped down, the hair follicles would be allowed to work normally. A side effect of cyclosporin, a drug that has to be taken for life by patients who have had an organ transplant (to stop rejection of the organ by the immune system), is extra hair growth – which suggests there could be something in this theory. However, taking cyclosporin by mouth could be extremely dangerous – laying the patient open to potentially fatal infection (even for transplant patients, there is a fine balance between over and under immune suppression).[8]

Chapter 9

The best of the rest

If you've decided against wigs, surgery, or drugs don't give up on your hair (or lack of it) quite yet. There are many other remedies, from acupuncture and herbs, to electrical treatments and nutritional therapy. Maybe there is something out there that will help with your hair loss.

Complementary medicine

In the UK, one person in four has consulted a complementary practitioner at some time in their lives, usually for an ailment which is hard to treat successfully with conventional medicine, such as back pain or chronic fatigue. Most systems of complementary medicine have specific therapies for treating hair loss (see table 8 below). There is insufficient space here to consider them all in detail, but some further information is given at the end of this chapter.

TABLE 8

Complementary therapies used in treatment of hair loss:

Acupuncture	Aromatherapy
Colour therapy	Counselling
Healing	Herbalism
Homeopathy	Hypnotherapy
Massage	Nutritional therapy
Polarity therapy	Psychotherapy
Reflexology	Traditional Chinese medicine

Complementary medicine usually adopts a 'whole person' approach, so seeing a practitioner may do some good on many levels. At the very least, you should benefit from a powerful placebo effect. Spending an hour or so on a regular basis with someone who is interested in you may be far more therapeutic than ten minutes with your overworked GP, waiting several months to see a dermatologist, or rubbing Regaine® into your scalp twice a day for the rest of your life. You may even grow back your hair (although – and this cannot be repeated too often – nothing is guaranteed. Steer clear of any therapist who says anything different).

Aromatherapy

The use of essential oils derived from plants stimulates the blood circulation and helps with drainage of toxins via the lymphatic system. You can use aromatherapy oils yourself, but do buy a good quality brand such as Nelson and Russell, Culpeper or Natural by Nature. They are available in most health food shops and at Boots. The oils listed in Table 9 are supposed to be particularly effective in improving the blood supply to the follicles, and in improving the circulation generally.

The oils can be used singly, or in combination. For a massage oil that can be used as a body rub, use five drops of oil to 10 ml of a 'carrier' oil such as sweet almond or jojoba. In a bath, use 4-6 drops of oil. A simple tip is to add one drop of rosemary to a final cold water rinse every time you wash your hair. This is said to stimulate the blood supply to the hair follicles.

Aromatherapist Valerie Worwood recommends the following mixture for hair loss: 2 drops cinnamon, 4 drops cypress, 4 drops geranium, 2 drops juniper, 5 drops lavender and 3 drops of rosemary. Mix one drop of the mixture with a quarter teaspoon of water and massage it into the scalp every night.

The Body Shop Reviving Aromatherapy Scalp Oil (£3.00 for 60mL), which is for weekly application, contains similar ingredients.

A clinical aromatherapist will be able to offer advice on self-help and give professional massage treatments. As discussed in chapter 4, massage alone is known to be beneficial to the hair and scalp. Done with aromatherapy oils, the results may be better still.[0]

TABLE 9

Aromatherapy oils which may help in case of hair loss

Basil	Cedar
Cypress	Geranium
Ginger	Grapefruit
Hyssop	Lavender
Lemon	Neroli
Rosemary	Sage
Thyme	

WARNING: Although aromatherapy oils are natural products, this does not mean they are without some medical risk. Do not use the following oils if you are, or think you might be, pregnant: basil, hyssop, juniper, sage and thyme. If you have epilepsy, you should not use hyssop or sage.

Herbs and Homeopathy

The use of herbs in medicine is probably as old as human history. Although herbal medicine has been overtaken by synthetic drugs over the last 100 years or so, many of these have a plant origin. And increasing numbers of people are turning to herbal remedies for a range of ailments, including hair loss.

English herbalist Nicolas Culpeper (1616-1654) produced a textbook of medicinal herbs, many of which are in use today, although not always for Culpeper's original indication. The aptly named golden maidenhair, for instance, can be boiled in water and used as a rinse to prevent thinning hair.

Southernwood, a common garden plant, is said to encourage hair growth. The dried herb should be added to rosemary, and used as a hair rinse after shampooing.

One herbal remedy which has hit the headlines recently is fenugreek, a common ingredient of curry powder and curry paste.

Known irreverently as 'the Balti cure', fenugreek is available commercially in capsule form as Arcon Tisane. You can also buy an accompanying lotion and shampoo. All the Arcon products also contain vitamins and minerals. The Arcon formula has been on sale in Germany and Scandinavia for some time, but has only recently been launched in Britain. It is available in hair salons, chemists shops, or by mail order (details at the end of this chapter). Prices are around £35 for a month's supply of capsules, while the shampoo is just over £11 and the lotion £15.00.[11]

Haar Sana is a range of hair products developed by Swiss herbalist Charles Vollrath over 50 years ago. The shampoo, conditioner and scalp lotion contain 27 Alpine herbs, including gentian, stinging nettle, alpine horsetail, burdock and camomile. The products are based on millet, a grain which is rich in silicon, which is a mineral important in keeping the hair in good condition. Millet shampoo costs about £5, conditioner is slightly more and the lotion for hair loss called Super Activator is just over £10 – all prices for a 200 mL bottle. They are available from health food shops, chemists or by mail order from the number given below.

There are several homeopathic remedies for hair loss, but if you want to try them you would be advised to consult a homeopath rather than treat yourself. Each remedy is meant to treat a 'whole body' condition rather than just one symptom, so the homeopath will want to diagnose you on this basis. For example, premature baldness and greying might be treated with Lycopodium, while hair loss with an itchy scalp often calls for Alumina. Homeopathic calcium is also said to give good results.[12]

Hypnotherapy

Where stress is a factor in hair loss, hypnotherapy can 'work wonders' says Deirdre Edwards, a member of the National Register of Hypnotherapists. She has helped several women with alopecia areata or telogen effluvium. Usually the hair loss can be traced back to repressed emotion from a childhood incident. Edwards guides her clients into a hypnotic state and encourages them to release the negative emotion. She then 'gets the hair moving again' by suggestion therapy, where they visualise their hair growing once more.

Six to eight weekly sessions are often all that are required to initiate regrowth. Often the hair will come back in the order it was lost. Once hair has started to grow, the client will return at fortnightly or monthly intervals for a 'top up' session. Between sessions they use an individualised relaxation tape which Edwards prepares for them, and work on building self esteem.

Edwards is not sure whether hypnosis would work for genetic hair loss, but thinks it may be worth a go if the client is in the early stages.[1, 3]

Nutrition-based therapies

The orthodox medical view is that you would get sufficient nutrients for your hair from a normal, balanced diet. The dietary ingredients that are most important for the hair have already been discussed in chapter 4. However, a growing number of people believe that vitamin and mineral deficiencies and/or food allergies or intolerance may lie at the root of many chronic ailments, including hair loss. If you are one of these, then read on.

As explained in chapter 2, hair loss in women can be due to an imbalance in the male/female sex hormone ratio. Stephen Davies and Alan Stewart (both medically qualified, which many nutritional therapists are not) suggest in their book 'Nutritional Medicine' that vitamin C and E supplementation may help shift the balance in the right direction in such cases. One gram of vitamin C a day is said to enhance the effect of oestrogens, while 600 IU (900 mg) Vitamin E a day may decrease the effect of male sex hormones.

There is no danger in taking this amount of vitamin C, but 600 IU is nearly 100 times the recommended daily allowance; supplementation at this level could cause some toxic effects. It may cause bleeding in people who are on anti-coagulant drugs and so should not be taken without close medical supervision. The importance of zinc in hair loss has already been discussed in chapter 4.[10]

Many of the products already mentioned contain vitamins and minerals in their formulation. In addition, there are others in which the vitamin/mineral is the main active ingredient. An example is Silicium 44, manufactured by the French company Laboratoires Carilene for women suffering hair loss due to the Pill or at menopause.

Silicium 44 contains organic silicon and is applied as a lotion to the scalp once a day at night time. The company has carried out several research trials in men and women with genetic hair loss. In the most recent, 90 people used the lotion for several months.

The investigators examined hair samples before and after the trial and showed that the proportion of hairs in the anagen (growing) phase increased in 87 per cent of cases. Silicium 44 also increases the diameter of the hair, giving better scalp coverage. Once the hair loss has been arrested, treatment can be discontinued. Silicium 44 is only available from Boots and costs about £20 for a 70 mL bottle (one month's supply). The accompanying shampoo costs£7.95 for a 150mL bottle.[2]

If you prefer to pop a pill rather than rub in a lotion, you could try a formula designed to support the skin and the connective tissue beneath the skin in an effort to revive the fortunes of your scalp. Advisors at Biocare, a company specialising in vitamins, herbs and minerals, admit the difficulty of treating hair problems and suggest trying their CT 241 or Colleginase supplements. CT 241 contains vitamin C, kelp – which is rich in many minerals – and horsetail, a source of silicon. Colleginase contains similar ingredients plus rutin and hesperidin which aid circulation in the capillaries beneath the skin. BioCare products are available by mail order from the number given below.

There is also MaxiHair (by Nature's Best, £12.95 for 60 tablets) which is a good basic supplement for thinning hair (NutriHair, also by Nature's Best is discussed in chapter 4).

Nourkrin also contains silicon, but its main active ingredients are compounds of marine origin, including an extract of a specific shark cartilage. It was developed in Finland after experiments on the use of shark cartilage extracts to renew aged and sun-damaged skin in women. Some of the women reported new hair growth, as well as beneficial effects on their skin. The product used in these trials is now available as Vivida (Nourella in the UK). Nourkrin comes as tablets, and can also be applied to the scalp as a lotion and a shampoo[7] In one published trial of Nourkrin for genetic hair loss, 40 young men (aged between 20 and 30) with hair loss on Hamilton scale III-V (Figure 3) were divided into two equal groups. One took two tablets of Nourkrin per day, while the other received placebo tablets made from fish extract. The investigators carried out hair counts on a small area of bald scalp at two, four and six months after the start of the trial. At six months, the Nourkrin group had an increase of 38 per cent in terminal hair, compared to only 2 per cent in the control group. At this stage, 19 out of 20 of the Nourkrin group were said no longer to have alopecia. The full results of the trial are given in Table 10.

Nourkrin has also been tested for alopecia areata. Ninety seven people from the Swedish Alopecia Association, who had tried many other treatments without success, enrolled in a 12 month study, with 83 of them completing the trial (the rest dropped out after three to four months because of lack of early effect). All took two tablets of Nourkrin per day. Fifty of the patients had alopecia areata, 12 alopecia totalis, and the remaining 21 had alopecia universalis.

At the end of the 12 month period, 7 out of 50 of the areata patients had 100 per cent regrowth, while 88 per cent claimed at least half their hair to have returned. Three out of 12 in the totalis group had 100 per cent regrowth, with three quarters counting more than 50 per cent. None of the universalis group showed complete hair regrowth, although 30 per cent showed regrowth of half their hair, or better.

The regrowth was estimated by the patients themselves (definitely a weak point as far as traditional clinical research is concerned) but the results were analysed by two independent

TABLE 10

Clinical trial of Nourkrin in men with genetic hair loss

Time in months		Nourkrin (20 patients)	Placebo (20 patients)
0	Av. hair counts	1238	1233
2		1318	1230
4		1419	1257
6		1710	1259

Haircounts are for an area of scalp of 2.5 cm diameter

dermatologists. A bonus was that all those with weak nails (which often occurs in alopecia areata) noticed stronger growth on Nourkrin.[17, 18]

Nourkrin has at least one famous fan. Film director Michael Winner swears by Nourkrin tablets, but also uses Regaine® and Philip Kingsley's scalp treatment (for details of these see chapters 8 and 4). Nourkrin is available from Selfridges (London), hair salons, health food shops and chemists. It is also available by mail order (address and phone number below). It costs about £45 per box of 60 tablets (one month's supply), around £20 for a 75ml bottle of lotion while the shampoo is £8.50 for a 150 ml bottle.

Traditional Chinese Medicine

Clinics and shops offering herbal remedies from Traditional Chinese Medicine (TCM) are springing up all over the UK. Used in the East for thousands of years, TCM is now gaining increasing recognition in the West.

Shen Min (which contains the ingredient, He Shou Wu, meaning 'black hair') is a Chinese herbal remedy for hair loss which has recently been launched here. In TCM, hair loss is seen as reflecting imbalances in the blood and the kidneys. Shen Min is said to act at this level. It is mentioned in standard Chinese medical works going back 400 years and is traditionally used to slow down the ageing process, which includes hair loss and greying. Shen Min is taken in tablet form 3 or 4 times a day. A modern clinical study of 822 patients with alopecia areata, carried out in China, suggested that 630 of them showed some hair regrowth after three months treatment.[6]

Shen Min is available from some health food shops, or from the contact number given below.

Figure 8: Exercises which increase blood flow to the scalp

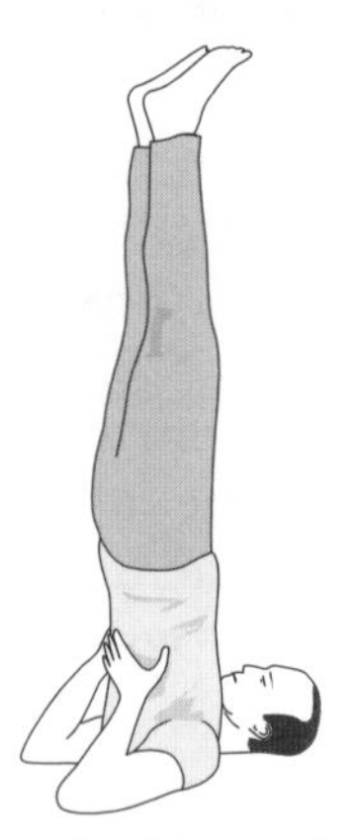

1 Yoga shoulder stand.

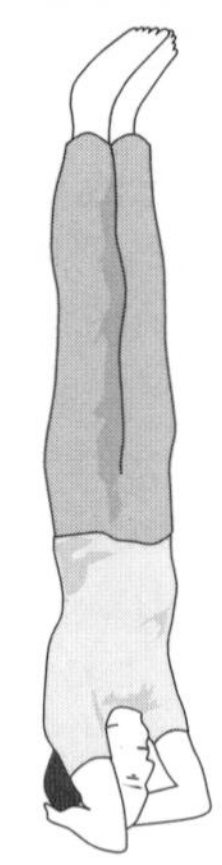

2 Yoga head stand (for experienced practitioners only).

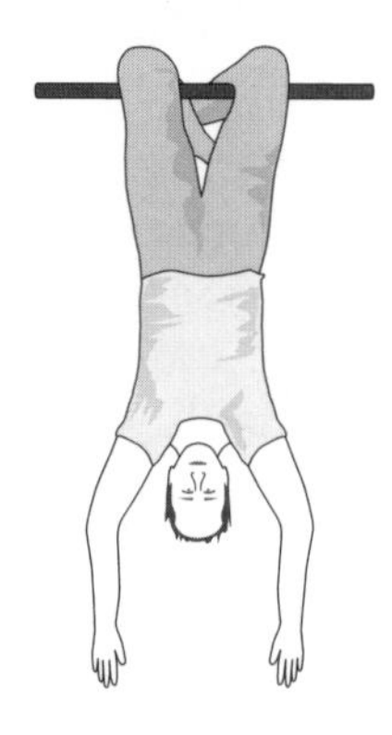

3 Hanging from a bar. Hook your knees over a parallel bar and let your body hang limp.

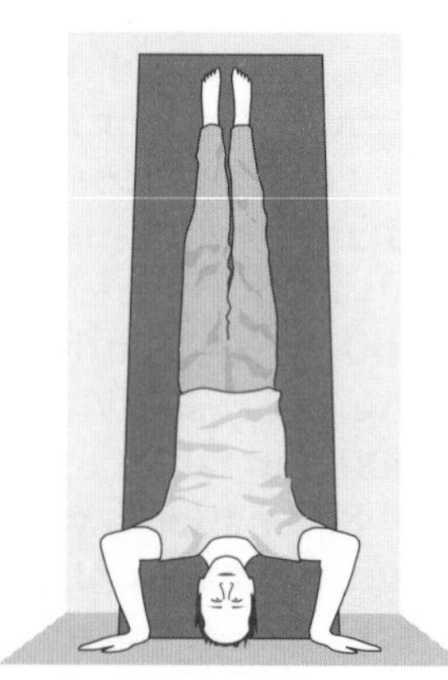

4 Inverting yourself on a board. Prop a board, the same length as your body, at a steep angle against a wall, and lie on it head downwards.

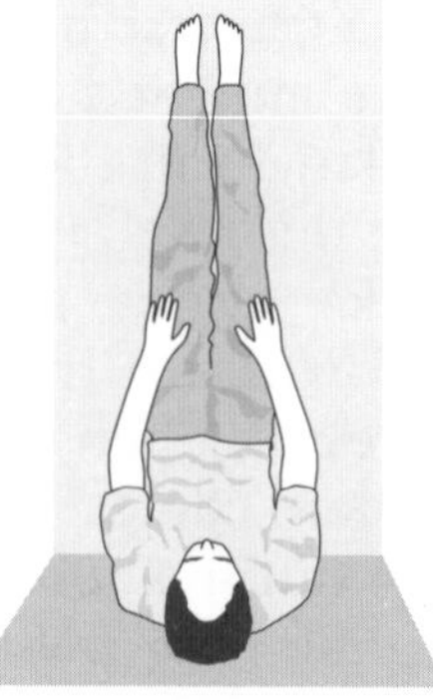

5 Feet against the wall. Lie on the floor with your legs up a wall, and rest your hands on your thighs.

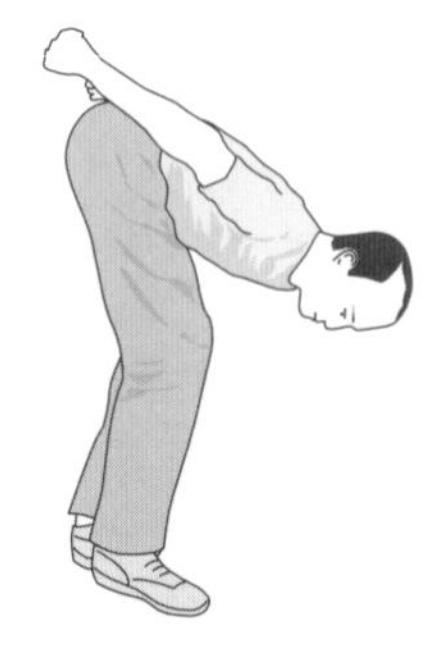

6 Bending over. Bend your head towards your toes; clasp your hands and raise them behind you.

Hanging upside down

Andy Bryant, author of a book provocatively titled '*The Baldness Cure*', believes that stress impairs the blood supply to the follicles and it is this, rather than the direct action of dihydrotestosterone, which is the cause of hair loss. Without a healthy blood supply, the follicles are starved of nutrients, and toxic waste products build up. There is certainly some evidence that scalp blood flow is impaired in genetic hair loss, so there may be something in Bryant's theory although most hair professionals scoff at it.[4, 8, 16]

The link between stress and changes in blood flow is well established. When you get stressed, the hormone adrenaline marshals several different physiological changes which put the body on full alert for a 'fight or flight' response. One of these responses is vasoconstriction, a narrowing of the blood capillaries beneath the skin, including the scalp. This diverts blood from the skin to the muscles, supplying them with extra energy to deal with the perceived threat. People under stress also carry chronic muscle tension in their neck, shoulders and scalp. The main scalp muscles actually lie above the eyes, above the ears and towards the back of the head. The rest of the scalp is covered with a sheet of fibrous tissue called aponeurosis, a tendon-like material which connects the muscles together. Bryant points out that the distribution of muscle and aponeurosis closely resembles the characteristic pattern of male pattern baldness. When scalp, neck and shoulder muscles contract under stress, he argues, they pull on the aponeurosis and this further cuts of blood supply to the follicles in this area.

The main feature of Bryant's 'cure' is the Inverter, a device which allows you to hang upside down, thus restoring the blood supply to the follicles. It is designed so that you lean back and control the degree of inversion with your arms.

Inversion causes the blood pressure to rise, and the body

compensates by opening up the capillaries under the skin, including the scalp – effectively reversing vasoconstriction. You begin by inverting to an angle of around 45 degrees to the vertical for around 30 seconds, morning and night and then work up to 90 degrees, gradually increasing the time, over a period of weeks to three minutes or so. Ex-Labour MP Bryan Gould apparently re-grew 50 per cent of his hair by inverting regularly.

However, the Inverter costs around £400. Cheaper alternatives include a number of simple exercises which get the feet above the head (see Figure 8). Note that inversion is not recommended if you suffer from high blood pressure, heart disease, and a number of other conditions. If in doubt, check with your doctor.

The inverter is the mainstay of a complete hair restoration programme run by Bryant's company Natural Hair Products. Other recommendations include:

❑ a high water content diet rich in fruit, vegetables and salad, preferably organic

❑ increasing your intake of filtered or mineral water to up to 2 litres a day

❑ relaxation exercises specifically for the shoulders, neck and scalp to be done morning and night

❑ use of stress monitors; these are tiny plastic dots which you stick on the inside of your wrist. They change colour as the temperature of the skin changes which in turn is a measure of the level of vasoconstriction accompanying stress. A high stress level goes with a lowered skin temperature (monitor colour black). As you relax, the capillaries dilate and the temperature rises. The monitor changes colour from black, through green, brown, to blue (very relaxed).

Along with all this goes plenty of sensible advice about long term stress management, which does not differ much from that available in any other self-improvement book. Also on offer is a urine test; this is meant to diagnose any vitamin or mineral deficiency which could be affecting your hair. The company will then supply you with various nutritional supplements. At the time of writing the full programme is on offer for £49.95 a month (details at the back of this book). Even if you grew no hair back at all, your general health would be almost certain to benefit from the Natural Hair Products dietary and stress management programme alone (you might even stop worrying about your hair). Having said that,much of this information is available elsewhere free of charge (just borrow the relevant books from your local library – some suggestions are made at the end of this chapter).

Andy Bryant is also associated with the Hair-Growers Club, which offers an annual £10,000 prize to the Hair-Grower of the Year and has a quarterly newsletter. Some people may find this group approach fun and helpful (just as many dieters say Weight Watchers helps motivate them).

James Oldham, 52, a sales executive from Henley, and winner of the Hair Grower's Prize in 1996, describes how the programme works in practice.

"I first started losing hair in my late 30s, and I'd lost a fair amount by the time I heard about Andy's programme – a year and a half before the Hair Grower's competition. It appealed because it sounded so logical. At the time I had a bad back and I thought the inverter would help that, though I wasn't sure I would grow back hair. But after only a week or so I was washing my hair in the bath and I noticed that much less was falling out - this made me feel a lot happier.

After about three months, my wife thought I was actually growing hair though it was fuzzy and colourless. Later on it came through dark. I was so encouraged that I stepped up my efforts. Someone said I'd a good chance of winning the competition and that really got me interested. The prize was a big incentive. I was measured and checked when I entered. By the time I'd won (after 18 months on the programme) my bald patch was reduced to around a third of its original size and I'd say I'd regained about half of the hair I'd lost.

So I think you can regrow your hair using Andy's method but you do have to put some effort into it. You may need to alter your lifestyle. I changed my diet completely. It's been very valuable to step up my water intake – I drink one and a half litres of filtered water a day and it's made a difference to all sorts of things. I eat more fruit and vegetables, and lots of salads. If I cook them at all, I'll steam them. And I don't eat pre-packaged food. I go for organic when I can afford it. I also exercise using a rebounder which gets the blood circulating. The benefits are I don't get colds or headaches any more.

My back pain has gone, I sleep better and I'm fitter. And my receding hairline is still improving. A lot of people get neurotic about losing their hair and I think it's great – especially for younger people – that there's hope for them, if they're prepared to make the necessary changes.

Nowadays, I believe the programme is tailor-made to the individual, with emphasis on targetted mineral/vitamin/herbal supplements, as well as the stress management and other standard aspects of the course. Anyone starting Andy Bryant's programme now should see even faster results."

ElectroTrichoGenesis (ETG)

It is an established medical fact that electric fields can speed up wound healing and the repair of bone fractures. Now electric field treatment is being used to stimulate hair growth. In 1990, researchers at the University of British Columbia published the first double-blind clinical trial of ElectroTrichogenesis (ETG) on men with alopecia androgenetica. Fifty six men with hair loss of grade III and IV on the Hamilton Scale (see Figure 4) were divided into treatment and control groups. Each received either ETG or a simulation of ETG for 12 minutes each week for 36 weeks (except for twice weekly treatments at the beginning, middle and end of the treatment period). At the end of this time, hair counts were up 66 per cent in the treatment group and 26 per cent in the control group. What is more, 29 out of 30 men in the treatment group showed either regrowth or no further hair loss.[13]

These results have since been confirmed by larger trials. None of the men involved in the trials reported any side effects from the process.[5]

ETG treatment involves sitting under a device similar to a salon hood-style hair dryer. The hair should be thoroughly dry beforehand. Nothing touches the scalp. The treatment is completely painless and appears to be absolutely safe.

Independent calculations show that you would need an electric field 100,000 times stronger than that used in ETG to induce an electric current in the body.

No-one is quite sure how ETG works. One theory is that the electric field causes the mineral calcium to enter cells in the papilla, giving a biochemical signal that makes them divide faster. ETG is being developed by the Canadian company Current Technology and is available, at the present time, in Canada, Australia, New Zealand, Mexico, India and the Philippines. It is set to arrive in the UK in the near future.[14]

More information

Books

Natural Therapies: The complete A-Z of complementary health, ed Margot McCarthy, Thorsons, £8.99

The Fragrant Pharmacy: A home and health care guide to

aromatherapy and essential oils, Valerie Ann Worwood, Macmillan, £16.95

Nutritional Medicine, Stephen Davies and Alan Stewart, Pan, £8.99

The Book of Stress Survival, Alix Kirsta, Gaia Books

The Stress Management Kit, Alix Needham, Virgin, £14.99 (contains stress sensor dots, a relaxation tape and a book)

Contacts

Arcon-Tisane is available by mail order from 01327-260393

For information on Haar Sana products & Shen Min contact 0171-435-5911

The National Council for Hypnotherapy, Hazelwood, Broadmead, Sway, Lymington, Hants, SO41 6DH Tel:01590-683770, will put you in touch with Deirdre Edwards or another therapist if you are considering hypnotherapy for your hair loss problem

Biocare mail order: tel 0121-433-3727

Nourkrin is available by mail order from Pharmavita Ltd PO Box 3379 London SW11 3ED Tel:0171-223-1665

For information about the Natural Hair Products programme, and the Hair Growers Club contact Andy Bryant on 01483-725702

Chapter 10

In the pipeline

There may well be an effective cure for genetic hair loss within the next few years. A number of approaches are being actively explored by drug companies and range from more sophisticated anti-androgens to gene-based therapies. There is also hope for those with alopecia areata as researchers gain new insights into the causes of this puzzling disorder.

5-alpha reductase inhibitors

It is pretty well established that the prime cause of genetic hair loss is an inherited over-sensitivity of the hair follicles to the male hormone dihydrotestosterone (DHT) (see chapter 2).

Since DHT is produced from the male sex hormone testosterone by the action of 5-alpha reductase, drugs which block (or inhibit) the action of this enzyme could, in theory, restore the normal function of the hair follicles.

There is already one 5-alpha reductase inhibitor on the market. Finasteride (Proscar) is a newish drug which is used in the treatment of benign prostatic hyperplasia (BPH), a condition in which the prostate becomes enlarged, leading to troublesome urinary symptoms. BPH is very common, particularly among older men. Dihydrotestosterone appears to be responsible for the enlargement of the prostate gland. Finasteride reduces DHT levels and causes the prostate to shrink back to a normal size.

Experiments in which balding stumptail macaque monkeys were given oral finasteride showed it to be about as effective as minoxidil in reducing hair loss. Analysis of the monkeys' hair showed that many telogen (resting) follicles had been converted into the anagen (growing) phase. When minoxidil and finasteride were used together, the effect seemed to be additive, with the monkeys growing more hair than they did with either drug used alone.

However, when topical finasteride was tried in a group of five men the results were disappointing; although the drug lowered DHT levels by about 40 per cent, none of the men regrew any hair.[3] The problem is that finasteride is not specific enough to the hair follicle. It turns out there are two forms of 5-alpha reductase. The type-I enzyme is active in the hair follicle, while the type-II enzyme is active in the prostate. Finasteride probably acts mainly on the type-II 5-alpha reductase. What is needed is a drug which is specific to the type-I enzyme that will just target the hair follicles.[2, 3]

Finasteride does not alter testosterone levels – an important consideration, as this could give rise to feminising side effects. However, a minority of men using finasteride suffer from impotence, reduced sex drive and reduced volume of semen when they ejaculate. And finasteride should never be taken by women of child-bearing age, as it can cause foetal deformities. Men taking it are advised to use condoms for intercourse as the drug finds its way into semen.

Further research is being carried out on finasteride.

While it may never be licensed as a treatment for genetic hair loss, it is still a very important 'lead' for the development of related drugs which will act as specific type-1 5-alpha reductase inhibitors.

Saw palmetto, the active ingredient of Prostatan (a herbal tincture manufactured by Bioforce), is also a 5-alpha reductase inhibitor. However, Prostatan is not known to have any effect upon hair loss. Zinc is also said to have some activity as a 5-alpha reductase inhibitor as is a plant extract known as pygeum.

Oestrogen blocking drugs

The female sex hormone oestrogen appears to play an important role in the hair cycle, according to new research carried out by scientists at North Carolina State University. Robert Smart and colleagues shaved the hair from the backs of female mice and applied 17-beta-oestradiol (a type of oestrogen) to the skin of one group, and a cream which blocks the effects of oestrogen to a second group. After two weeks of treatment, the first group remained bald, while the hair on the second group had grown back to the same thickness as before shaving. It looks as if topical oestrogen locks the hair into the telogen (resting) phase, while the oestrogen blocker shifts it back into the anagen (growth) phase. This fits with the observation that pregnant women, who have high levels of oestrogen, replace plucked hair more slowly than women who are not pregnant.

Smart is now planning to repeat these experiments in humans; if he finds oestrogen is important in the human hair cycle, then an oestrogen blocking cream could be developed for treating hair loss. It is not yet clear what kind of hair loss such a drug might be useful for.[4, 5]

Growing hair in a test tube

In 1990, Terence Kealey and Michael Philpott of Cambridge University discovered how to make human hair grow in test tubes (or in vitro, to use the technical term). Using hair follicles from skin samples left over from face-lift operations, they carefully 'planted' each one in a nutrient solution in a tiny sample tube. By experimenting with the nutrients, they were eventually able to get the hair to keep growing for 10 days, at the same rate as it does on a human head. By 1994, they had even worked out how to grow hair with the sebaceous glands attached.[6-9]

Kealey and Philpott's work is backed by the multinational

chemical giant Unilever. The company stands to make a good return on its investment, for the in vitro system opens the door to the discovery of the elusive factors which make hair grow, or – even more important – stop it from growing. Already they have shown that, as you might expect, minoxidil strongly stimulates hair growth. A group of naturally occurring chemicals known as growth factors also appear to exert significant influence on the growth of hair follicles. One of these, known as epidermal growth factor (EGF) actually shifts hair from anagen to catagen, creating a club hair which is ready to be shed. This is in line with experiments on sheep; injections of EGF make them shed their fleece. Till then, EGF had mainly been known for its role in wound healing – for it speeds up the growth of new tissue beneath a scar. Another growth factor, transforming growth factor, has a similar effect to EGF. However, a third member of this group, insulin-like growth factor turns out to be a strong stimulator of hair growth.[10]

The immune system also plays a role in hair growth. A group of chemicals known as cytokines, which help the body to fight infection, also appear to inhibit the growth of the hair. It may be that people suffering from genetic hair loss and alopecia areata have some defect in the way their body produces and/or handles growth factors and cytokines. Drugs which can block or enhance the effects of these natural body chemicals are clear candidates for new and effective hair loss treatments.

Gene therapy for hair loss?

No-one knows which genes are important in hair loss. However, some people with alopecia areata have a different form of the gene for a substance called interleukin-1 receptor antagonist (IL-1 RA), compared to the rest of the population. Interleukin-1 is one of the cytokines mentioned above and IL-1 RA is involved in 'damping down' its effects on the body. If

IL-1 RA is not doing its job properly (and the above change in its gene suggests it may not be) then interleukin-1 gets out of control, possibly triggering an autoimmune attack on the hair follicles.

A second potential hair loss gene has come from experiments in mice. These particular mice began to go bald when they were 2 to 3 weeks old, and by the time they were six weeks old they had lost all their hair. It turned out that their gene for an enzyme called ornithine decarboxylase (ODC) was over-active. When the research team, based in Pennsylvania, blocked ODC with a drug called 2-difluoromethylornithine, the mice did not lose their hair. If people with hair loss also have a problem with ODC, then there is already a potential drug on offer.[11]

Since genetic hair loss tends to get worse with age, many hair experts wonder if it is just part and parcel of the ageing process. Uncovering the genes which are involved in ageing – currently a hot research topic – may provide new insights into why people lose their hair. And maybe some of the anti-ageing drugs which are currently being researched will also help people keep their hair.

Humans have between 50 and 100 thousand genes. There is currently an international effort, known as the Human Genome Project, whose aim is to identify each one of these genes – including, of course, those involved in the hair cycle. Once these genes are discovered, there will be two ways forward. First, inhibitor drugs which can block their action, if need be, can be designed. The second approach is gene therapy.

If someone has hair loss because one of their genes is faulty then they can be given a 'normal' copy. Gene therapy is already underway for cystic fibrosis, some rare immune disorders and for some forms of cancer.

The main problem in gene therapy is how to deliver the gene to the cells where it is needed. But Ligna Li and Robert

Hoffman of AntiCancer, a biotechnology company in California, have already shown that you can target genes specifically to the hair follicles. They grew hair in vitro and treated it with liposomes – a type of fatty droplet – containing a 'marker' gene. Cells that take up this 'marker' strain blue under the microscope. Li and Hoffman discovered that only the hair follicles, and not the surrounding skin, went blue. So in theory one day you could treat hair loss quite safely with a 'gene shampoo'.[12, 13]

Sources

1. Medline database search, 1990-1996

Chapter 1

2. *Human Anatomy & Physiology*, 3rd Edition, D. van Wynsberghe, C.R.Noback and R.Carola, Mc Graw Hill,1990

3. *Diseases of the Hair and Scalp*, ed Rook A & Dawber R, Blackwell, 1991

4. Rook, Wilkinson & Ebling's *Textbook of Dermatology*, 5th Ed, ed R.H.Chapman et al, Blackwells, 1992

5. *Bodywatching*, Desmond Morris, Grafton, 1985

Chapter 2

1. Interviews with John Firmage and Keith Hobbs at the Scalp & Hair Clinic, 108 St John's Hill, Clapham Junction, London SW11

2. Interview with Dr Hugh Rushton, 22 Harley St London W1

3.Biochemical and trichological characterisation of diffuse alopecia in women, D.H.Rushton et al, *Br J Dermatol* 123,1990, 187-19

4. Natural progression of male pattern baldness in young men, D.H.Rushton, *Clin Exp Dermatol*, 1991, 16,188-92

5. Life with alopecia totalis, *Dermatology in Practice*, 1996, Jan/Feb, 12-13

6. Chemotherapy-Induced Alopecia: New Developments, Atif M. Hussein, *Southern Medical Journa*l, 1993, 86, 489-494

7. Subcutaneous blood flow in early male pattern baldness, Per Klemp et al, *J Invest Dermatol*, 1989,92, 725-6

8. Alopecia: Diagnosis and management, *American Family Physician*, 1995, 51, 1513-1522

9. Management of hair loss in women, D.H.Rushton, *Dermatologic Clinics*, 1993, 1, 47-53

10. Investigating and managing hair loss in apparently healthy women, D.H.Rushton, *Canadian J Dermatol*, 5, 455-461

11.Hair loss in women: what to say and do to ease these patients' distress, *Postgraduate Medicine*, 1992, 91, 417-431

12.Premature grey hair and hair loss among smokers: a new opportunity for health education, J.G.Mosley and A.C.C.Gibbs, *British Medical Journal*, 1996, 313, 1616

13.Does stress make women go bald, Bonnie Estridge, *Daily Mail*, November 16, 1996

14. *Hair Loss: Coping with alopecia areata and thinning hair*, Elizabeth Steel, Thorsons1995

Chapter 3

1. Does fortune favour the bald? Psychological correlates of hair loss in males, Pamela A.Wells et al *Br J Psychol* 1995 86 337-344

2. Psychologic characteristics of men with alopecia androgentica and their modification, J. van der Donk et al, *Int J Dermatol* 1991 30 22-28

3. The psychological effects of androgenetic alopecia in men, T.F.Cash, *J Am Acad Dermatol*, 1992, 26, 926-931

4. *P*sychological problems with hair loss in general practice and the treatment policies of general practitioners, E.B.G.de Koning et al, *Psych Reports*, 1990, 67, 775-778

5. Individual differences in men's perceptions of and reactions to thinning hair, *J Soc Psych* 1989, 130, 209-218

6. Losing Hair, losing points? The effects of male pattern baldness on social impression formation, T.F.Cash, *J App Social Psych* 1990 20 154-167

7. Psychological effects of androgenetic alopecia on women: comparisons with balding men and with female control subjects, T.F.Cash, *J Am Acad Dermatol* 1993 29 568-575

Chapter 4

1. *Hair: An owner's handbook*, Philip Kingsley, Aurum Press, 1995

2. *Hairdressing Science*, 3rd Ed, Florence Openshaw, Longman 1995

3. The best cuts for thinning hair, Laura Bacharach, *Men's Health*, September 1996

4. Can a crash diet make you go bald? Bonnie Estridge, *Daily Mail*, December 10 1996

5. So you want thicker hair? Nadine Baggott, *Daily Mail*, December 9, 1996

6. Best cuts for thinning hair, Stephen Perrine, *Men's Health*, April/May 1995

Chapter 5

1. Interview with Caroline Woolfson on cold cap treatment during chemotherapy

2. *How to Complain*, Bridget Avison, Longman's Self-Help Guides, 1986

3. *You and Yours How to Complain*, David Berry, BBC Books, 1990,Trichology Clinics

4. Interview with Bill Lennon at the Advertising Standards Authority

5. Interview with Michelle Goddard in legal department of Consumers Association

Chapter 6

1. Interview with Richard Mawbey, Designer of Wig Specialities Ltd, 173 Seymour Place, London W1H 5TP Tel: 0171-262-6565 Fax:0171-723-1566

2. *Coping with Hair Loss*, booklet for cancer patients from BACUP, 3 Bath Place, Rivington St London EC2A 3JR Tel;0171-696-9003

3. Wigs for your patients, *Dermatology in Practice*, 1996, January/February p15

Chapter 7

1. Interview with Dr Michael May, Vice-President of the British Association of Hair Restoration Surgeons

2. *Hair Transplantation*, 3rd Ed, 1995, ed Walter P Unger

3. Hair replacement surgery for male pattern alopecia, D.Green et al, *Medical Clinics of North America*, 1993, 3 689-703

4. Hair to stay, Judy Sadgrove, *Men's Health*, April 1996

5. Puig Medical Group (http://www.pmghair.com/)

Chapter 8

1. Interview with Annabel-Fiddian Green, Vane Percy & Associates (PR for Pharmacia & Upjohn)

2. New treatments for alopecia areata, M Lebwohl, *Lancet*, 1997, 349

4. Five year follow up of men with androgenetic alopecia treated with topical minoxidil, E.A.Olsen et al, *J Am Acad Dermatol* 1990 22 643

6. Quantitative estimation of hair growth; comparative changes in weight and hair count with 5 per cent and 2 per cent minoxidil, placebo and no treatment, V.Price & E.Menefee, *Hair Research for the next Millennium*, 1996, 67, Elsevier

7. Reversal of baldness in patient receiving minoxidil for hypertension, A.R.Zappacosta, *NEJM* 1980 1480

8. Alopecia Areata: Update on therapy, *Dermatologic Clinics*, 1993 11 35

9. Topical minoxidil dose-response effect in alopecia areata,V.C.Fiedler-Weiss et al *Arch Dermatol* 1986 122 180

10. The importance of adequate serum ferritin levels during oral cyproterone acetate and ethinyl oestradiol treatment of diffuse androgen-dependent alopecia in women, D.H.Rushton & I.D.Ramsay, *Clinical Endocrinology*, 1992, 36, 421

11. Androgenetic alopecia in the female, R.D.DeVillez, *Arch Dermatol* 1994 130 303

12. Advances in alopecia areata and androgenetic alopecia, M.E.Sawaya & M.K.Hordinsky, *Adv Dermatol* 1992 7 211

13. Treatment of female androgenetic alopecia with minoxidil 2 per cent D.A.Whiting & Coleman Jacobson *Pharmacology &*

Therapeutics, 1992 11 800

14. Systemic steroids with or without 2 per cent topical minoxidil in the treatment of alopecia areata, E.A.Olsen et al *Arch Dermatol* 1992 128 1467

15. Minoxidil Update on its clinical role R.C.Savin & A.V. Atton, *Dermatologic Clinics*, 1993 11 55

Chapter 9

1. Interview with Deirdre Edwards, hypnotherapist

2. Interview with Tracey Hollom, PR for Carilene Labs, about Silicium 44

3. Success Story 'Hypnotherapy cured my hair loss' *Here's Health*, July 1996

4. Subcutaneous blood flow in early male pattern baldness, P.Klemp et al *J Invest Dermatol* 1989 92 725

5. Electrotrichogenesis: Further evidence of efficacy and safety on extended use, *Int J Dermatol* 1992 31 878

6. Jeri Trachtman, Biotech Corporation, Glastonbury CT Tel 860638-8111 for Chinese clinical studies on Shen Min

7. Nigel Fawkes, Pharmavita, for information on Nourkrin 0171-223-1665

8. Interview with Andy Bryant, author of *The Baldness Cure*, Vermilion, 1994

9. Valerie Worwood, *Aromatherapy*, Macmillan

10. Interview with John McLaren Howard (associate of Dr Stephen Davies, author of Nutritional Medicine) 0171-636-5959

11. Interview with Hitesh Patel, Arcon UK, 01733-66638 on fenugreek

12. *The Hamlyn Encyclopaedia of Complementary Health* for information on homeopathy

13. The Biological effects of a Pulsed Electrostatic field with specific reference to Hair, W.S.Maddin et al *Int J Dermatol* 1990 29 446

14. Interview with Anne Kramer of Current Technology, Vancouver,604 684 2727 on current status of electrotrichogenesis, (http://www.currentech.com/)

15. *Gone Today, Hair Tomorrow*, Maxim, August 1996

16. A comparative study of a new food supplement ViviScal, with fish extract for the treatment of hereditary androgenic alopecia in young males, A.Lassus and E.Eskelinen,*J Int Med Res*, 1992 20 445

17. Treatment of alopecia areata and alopecia totalis with Viviscal (marine derived polysaccharide, Nourkrin) A.Lassus et al submitted to*J Am Acad Dermatol*

18. Oral treatment of alopecia areata, alopecia totalis and alopecia universalis. A 12 month test of the food supplement ViviScal, *Swedish Association for Alopecia*

19 Interview with Karen Dye, Technical Support at BioCare, 0121-433-3727

Chapter 10

1. Hair growth effects of oral administration of finasteride, a steroid 5-alpha reductase inhibitor alone and in combination with topical minoxidil in the balding stumptail macaque, A.R.Diani et al,*J Clin Endocrinology*, 1992, 74,345-350

2. Dihydrotestosterone, W. Brink, Musclemag

3. Topical 0.05per cent finasteride significantly reduced serum DHT concentrations, but had no effects in preventing the expression of genetic hair loss in men, D.H.Rushton et al, *Hair Research for the next millennium*, 1996, 359-362

4. Controlling hair growth, *Chemistry & Industry*, 1996, 4th November, 817

5. An estrogen receptor pathway regulates the telogen-anagen hair follicle transition and influences epidermal cell proliferation, H-S Oh and R. Smart, *Proc Nat Acad Sci*, 1996, 93, 12525-12530

6. Prolonged maintenance of human hair follicles in vitro in a

serum-free medium, G.E.Westgate et al, *Br J Dermatol* 1993, 129,372-379

7. Effects of EGF on the morphology and patterns of DNA synthesis in isolated human hair follicles, M. P.Philpott and T. Kealey, *J Invest Dermatol*, 1994, 102,186-191

8. Human hair growth in vitro: a model for the study of hair follicle biology, M.P. Philpott et al *J Dermatol Sci* 1994, 7(Suppl) S55-S72

9. The isolation and maintenance of the human pilosebaceous unit, D.A.Sanders et al *Br J Dermatol* 1994 131 166-176

10. Cultured human hair follicles and growth factors, M.P.Philpott et al *J Invest Dermatol* 1995 104 (Suppl) 44S-45S

11. Modulation of murine hair follicle function by alterations in ornithine decarboxylase activity, A P Soler et al *J Invest Dermatol* 1996 106 1108-1113

12. Could 'gene shampoo' cure balding? Abi Berger, *New Scientist*, 1995, I July, 1

13. The feasibility of targeted selective gene therapy of the hair follicle, L.Li and R.M.Hoffman, *Nature Medicine*, 1995, 1, 705-706